The Art of Medicine

What Every Doctor and Patient Should Know

The Art of Medicine

What Every Doctor and Patient Should Know

A National Award-Winning Health Reporter and Emergency Physician provides invaluable insights into how to bring care and compassion to the doctor-patient relationship.

Kevin J. Soden, MD, MPH, FAAFP

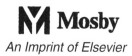

Mosby

An Imprint of Elsevier

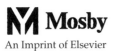
Mosby

An Imprint of Elsevier

The Cutis Center
Independence Square West
Philadelphia, PA 19106

NOTICE

Medicine is an ever-changing field. Standard safety precautions must be followed, but as new research and clinical experience broaden our knowledge, changes in treatment and drug therapy may become necessary or appropriate. Readers are advised to check the most current product information provided by the manufacturer of each drug to be administered to verify the recommended dose, the method and duration of administration, and contraindications. It is the responsibility of the licensed prescriber, relying on experience and knowledge of the patient, to determine dosages and the best treatment for each individual patient. Neither the publisher nor the editor assumes any liability for any injury and/or damage to persons or property arising from this publication.

The Publisher

International Standard Book Number 0-323-02369-X

Library of Congress Control Number: 2003103379

Printed in United States of America

Last digit is the print number: 9 8 7 6 5 4 3 2 1

Table of Contents

✣ Dedication ✣

To my wife, Meg, who not only supported me in this effort, but also provide many stories and insights from her own medical school days.

To all my family for all the love and support they have given me through the many months it took writing this book.

To all the wonderful physicians who, by word and by example, have taught and who practice the Art of Medicine with their patients.

✣ Acknowledgments ✣

Many doctors were important to the final manuscript. Some allowed me to interview them and gain from their experience and insights while others contributed by reading and critiquing part of the text. This book would not have been written without their help. I would like to thank: Dr. Robert Watson, Dr. Bernard Lown, Dr. Patrick Ober, Dr. J. Patrick O'Leary, Dr. Robert Rakel, Dr. Clifton Meador, Dr. Curt Tribble, Dr. John Nackashi, Dr. Doug Newburg, Dr. Jape Taylor, Dr. Joanne Stenger, Dr. Lewis Sigmon, Dr. William Porter, Dr. Joseph Talley and Dr. Stephanie Richter.

Thanks to Richard Zorab and Christine Dumas who helped with the all important beginning meetings with the publisher and support along the way. Nancy Payne provided advice and counsel with my early efforts.

Many special thanks to Amy Rodgers who provided many wonderful editing suggestions and insights about writing and preparing a final manuscript. Her confidence in me and advice along the way were invaluable for a first time writer.

Thanks to Joe Kulka for his many wonderful cartoons that support the text.

Finally, many thanks to Bill Schmitt, my publisher at Elsevier, who has been extremely supportive throughout the entire publishing process and most patient with a first time writer. His advice and guidance have helped to make this book better in many ways.

A Note from the Author

Where do medical students, residents, physician assistants, nurse practitioners and other healthcare professionals learn the **Art of Medicine?** Almost exclusively, it is learned through the role modeling done by the teachers they encounter in the classrooms, clinics and bedsides of academic medical centers. Unfortunately, there seems to be increasing concern with this system of learning the Art as judged by the consumers of healthcare . . . our patients. In survey after survey, the consumers of health care list the failure of their doctors to listen to them as their number one complaint about the care they've been given. So, what are the root causes behind this problem with patient care?

Unfortunately, there are many reasons for these problems. In recent years, the faculties of these academic medical centers have seen tremendous encroachments on the time they have available to teach our future doctors and healthcare providers. First, there are increased pressures on existing staff to generate income, due to significant decreases in funding from state and federal governments, as well as decreases in reimbursement from insurance companies and managed care organizations. Second, research remains an ongoing pressure for faculty as part of the "publish or perish" mentality in the academic world. These are probably the two biggest forces that impact the short-changing of young doctors' training, but certainly not all the reasons.

Technological advances seem to occur on almost a daily basis, and last year's MRI or CT scanner just doesn't have what is needed to make the correct diagnosis this year (or so the salesperson would have us believe). To paraphrase one of the great physician teachers of the past century, Sir William Osler, "There is so much to learn about the science and about disease that little time is left to learn about the patient with the disease." I apologize to Dr. Osler for changing his wording but, I hope, not the emphasis).

The single trend with the greatest negative impact on the time physicians have to spend with patients may be the rise of managed care organizations. Some might disagree with this statement but the perception by those in practice strongly supports this viewpoint. Fueled by reimbursement schemes such as HMO capitation, the last twenty-five years of clinical practice have seen a dramatic decrease in the time a physician can spend with patients. This is directly related to productivity demands, the increased use of clinical guidelines, utilization reviews of hospital admissions and "cookbook" medicine. These trends will likely not improve, so to learn the Art of Medicine we must work smarter—because we will not have the luxury of working longer.

In preparing to write this book, I reviewed recent medical books and journals to see what had been published on the Art of Medicine. I assumed (and we all know how dangerous this can be) that there would be a number of articles on the subject since there should be a great deal of interest in the Art. With few exceptions, there was almost *nothing* in our medical journals that pertained to the Art. There were several notable books published in the last fifteen years, and these attempted to provide insight into the interaction between doctor and patient. The biggest problem with these books is that they were geared primarily for physicians who were already in the practice of medicine. I believe that, with rare exception, it is too late to effect much change in these practicing physicians unless the physician is motivated by what Dr. Morris Massey describes as a "significant emotional event" in his or her life. This might be a death of a patient, a missed diagnosis, a personal illness, or, more likely, a lawsuit. The statement may sound cynical but this has been the case in my twenty-five years of practicing medicine.

Therefore this book is primarily intended for premedical students, medical students and residents, as well as other healthcare providers. It also may be useful to us as doctors in our roles as future patients (because we will all become patients sooner or later). As patients we all have an obligation to hold our physicians' feet to the fire by defining what we expect from our relationship with them, including the care we want for our loved ones and ourselves. By acting as educated consumers of medical care, we will help to teach physicians what is needed to be the best practitioners of the Art of Medicine. We can learn the science of medicine from many places, but learning the Art only comes from observing doctor-patient interactions that are characterized by honesty and openness and through positive and negative feedback.

To better reach my intended reading audience, I have put my message into story form. This format is easier to read and provides a method of learning about the Art that is somewhat Socratic (the teaching style that medical educators have used from earliest times). It's through stories that we gain the most insight into life. It's through the stories of our patients' lives that we learn the most about them so that we can be the most beneficial to them. I use the Advisor as the universal teacher and the Student as a surrogate for all of us who are constantly learning the Art of Medicine from our teachers and patients. I have tried to present the material in a style that is readable and provides some humor. The book also contains references to works by other physicians; these offer additional insight into the doctor-patient relationship and supplement my views on the subject. Included in each chapter is a section that provides special messages to further enhance the understanding of a particular subject as well as a different perspective.

Introduction

It was late Friday night and the local chapter of the knife and gun club had already begun to meet in the hospital's emergency room. Police cars and ambulances seemed to be arriving frequently at the ER's front doors. The noise level in the ER's waiting room seemed to be growing louder with every minute. Almost every square inch of space was taken as the Student was wheeled into one of the far corners of the room to wait until his swollen, discolored ankle could be evaluated.

He had been playing pickup basketball with some of the other medical students in their regular Friday night game when his foot had come down on another player's. His ankle turned violently. The popping sound that accompanied the injury was audible to everyone in the gym. The ankle began swelling immediately and he couldn't bear weight on it at all due to the pain. The Student's friends brought him to the ER, told him to call them on their cell phones when he was done, and they would come to collect him.

The clientele that filled the waiting room was a true cross section of society with people of all races, colors and creeds packed into a very small area. The Student could hear foreign languages being spoken, some recognizable, but most unfamiliar to him. He hoped that he wouldn't have to wait too long. He just didn't feel comfortable around people he didn't know and with whom he didn't appear to have much in common. He tried to focus on the baseball game that was on the TV in the corner of the waiting room. As he began to adjust to the clamor around him he found himself sporadically eavesdropping on some of the conversations taking place around him.

Two well-dressed, middle-aged women sat on the couch next to him and the one closest was speaking with great emotion, "You won't believe what happened to my friend the other day. She went to her doctor to get the results of some X-ray tests that had been ordered after her breast biopsy came back positive. First of all, she had the biopsy done. It took her doctor's office two days to call her back and all they told her was that the doctor wanted to go over the results with her. Could she come in two weeks later? She nearly went crazy on the phone. 'What do you mean two weeks? What were the results? What do you mean you won't tell me because your policy is only to tell people in person?' After ranting and raving, she got an appointment in three days. Can you imagine all that went through her mind during those three days? I would have been going crazy." The woman telling the story stopped and just shook her head in amazement.

"Well don't leave me in suspense. What happened next?" her friend asked. The Student couldn't help it but he found himself leaning closer so he could hear them better.

"She did see the doctor who told her that it looked like she had cancer of the breast and that the tumor needed to be removed. Before he would do that, he needed to do some other tests so that he could 'stage' the tumor. He told her this and then said that he'd send his nurse in to arrange all the tests for a few weeks later. Then he got up, left the room, and she never saw him again until a few weeks later when her tests were done. Can you imagine the state of shock she was in when he told her, 'You've got breast cancer'? I wouldn't have heard a thing after he said that. Then, the bastard just ups and leaves without giving her time to ask any questions. That was bad enough, but the worst part was that she had to wait two weeks before all the tests were done and he saw her again to give her the results. She was hysterical that entire time and all she could do was picture the most horrible scenarios. . . . and her with two young children. Frankly, I'd never go see that doctor again. He's got all the sensitivity of that wall over there."

The other woman interrupted. "Good God, Lois, don't leave me hanging. What finally happened to your friend?"

"The good news was that all her tests were negative. The tumor hadn't spread. She did have surgery but only needed a lumpectomy. They did get the entire tumor and the surgeon did an excellent job. Everyone says he's brilliant technically. You can hardly see a scar on my friend but I'd never go to him. Give me my doctor any day. He sits and actually carries on a conversation with me. I can ask questions. He really seems to care about me as a person. He's wonderful." She gushed with great enthusiasm.

Enough of that crap, the Student thought. *What's the big deal? She did fine and the doctor did a great job with her scar. Did she want someone who does a great surgery or someone to hold her*

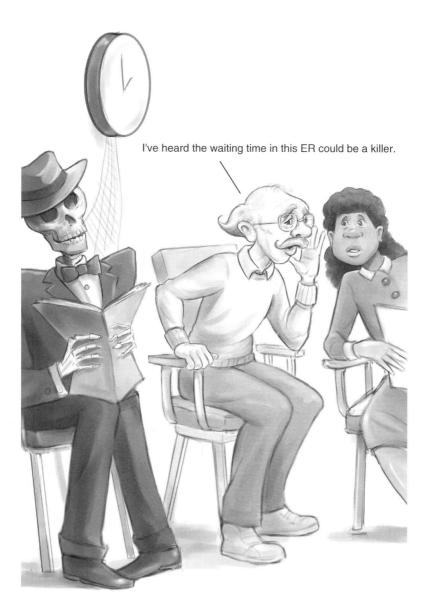

hand? Get a life! An angry voice suddenly interrupted his thoughts.

"I've been sitting here in this damn waiting room for five hours and I ain't heard one word from a damn soul about when I'm goin' to be seen. This is no way to treat people," said a large woman sitting one row over.

The much older man sitting next to her replied, "Sister, you are sooo right. I've waited so long in waiting rooms that I could've gone to medical school." They both laughed hilariously at their little joke and the Student found himself smiling despite himself.

A younger woman sitting across from them said, "I know it's busy here in this ER but all it would take would be for someone to come out regularly and tell us what the situation is and how long they think it might take for them to get to the minor problems. I know that all I've got is a urinary tract infection but I've got no regular doctor and nowhere else to go."

The other couple nodded in sympathy and then the woman said, "Honey, I agree with you. Why can't people learn to be more courteous? I waited in my doctor's office the other day for two hours, and I had an appointment. You've got to do better than that. Can you imagine if you made people wait like that at a restaurant and they had a reservation— and then no one ever said anything to them the whole time they were waiting? Do you think you'd ever go back to that place again? You could bet your sweet you-know-what that I never would." Everyone just laughed but it was only temporary relief for the frustration and injustice they were all feeling.

The Student thought about responding but decided it wasn't his problem. He thought they were just lucky to be able to see a doctor in the ER. He really didn't understand why they didn't have a regular doctor of their own. Again, his thoughts were interrupted but this time it was because the nurse was calling his name. It was his turn to be seen. He had a higher priority than the others around him because of the concern that his ankle might be broken. Unseen to him as he was wheeled into the ER, three more patients took his place in the waiting room. It was going to be another long, busy night in the emergency room.

✣ *Perspectives for Doctors* ✣

Medicine is considered both an art and a science. The Art of Medicine is so simple and yet so complex that it defies definition. Most would agree that the Art is what happens between a doctor and a patient that cannot be found in a scientific text. This interaction requires a physician to possess compassion, understanding, and sympathy, while being both supportive and emotionally available. It requires strong communication skills and great listening skills. The requirements are enough to intimidate the best men and women.

Unfortunately, recent years have seen the emphasis in the education of future physicians shift so that the time devoted to the Science of medicine has far surpassed that devoted to the Art. Medical school curricula pay scant attention to the Art while residency-training programs for the most part ignore the Art of Medicine except for what is learned from the rare teacher who might model it at the bedside. The impetus for this change in emphasis has been brought about by a number of factors. Chief among them are the tremendous advances in medical knowledge in both the basic sciences and the clinical disciplines

In most cases, the diagnosis and treatment of a patient depend on the physician's ability to gather and exchange information with the patient. Patient satisfaction and improved patient outcomes are clearly related to enhanced communication and listening skills on the part of physicians. On the negative side, poor communication between physician and patient was identified as the single most common cause for malpractice suits in a recent *Maryland Medical Journal* article. The very real fear of being sued that has been fueled by spurious suits and unrealistic patient expectations has led to a tremendous increase in unnecessary testing and more reliance on technology.

When researchers studied how physicians arrived at a diagnosis in their patients, they found that **history taking alone accounted for the correct diagnosis almost 70% of the time.** The laboratory and the hands-on exam only led to a diagnosis in the remaining 30% of cases. These data further strengthen the need for physicians skilled in effectively communicating with their patients. Likewise, the more thorough the history and clinical examination, the more focused and cost effective can be the subsequent laboratory or radiological evaluation.

The bottom line: It's all about taking care of people in a way that enables doctors or healthcare professionals to hear patients' stories and learn of their concerns, so that mind-body-spirit health problems can be addressed in a caring, compassionate manner.

Beginning the Art of Medicine and Finding Your Dream

"Not much happens without a dream. And for something great to happen, there must be a dream. Behind every great achievement is a dreamer of great dreams. Much more than a dreamer is required to bring it to reality; but the dream must be there first."

–Robert Greenleaf,
Servant Leadership

The Medical Student peered cautiously through the open door into the dimly lit interior of the office. The only light in the office came from a small desk lamp and a computer screen. The Student's Advisor had his back to him and was typing on the computer's keyboard with an awkward non-traditional style that seemed to require an aggressive pounding approach along with an almost constant stream of unintelligible mutterings to himself. The Medical Student waited for a minute before reaching around to knock timidly on the door.

"Come on in, Student, and have a seat. Oh, loosen that tie of yours and get comfortable while you're at it," said the

Advisor without turning in his chair. "I'll be with you in a minute. I need to finish this one e-mail to a patient of mine."

The Student slowly entered and sat in the rather comfortable high-backed chair next to the Advisor's desk. He chose not to loosen his tie, since he thought it would make a better impression. The Student hoped the meeting wouldn't take too long as he wanted to get back downstairs to see a relatively new radiology procedure. But first he had to meet his Advisor, who was also to serve as his mentor for learning something the medical school called the Art of Medicine.

Art. Schmart. Whatever, the Student thought irritably. *This is a waste of my time when I could be downstairs where the action is, learning how to really heal people.*

He'd come to medical school with the dream of becoming an interventional radiologist, and some of the courses that he had to take to get to this goal were absolutely ridiculous. This Art of Medicine one was a perfect example.

What a joke! This is one hour a week of my valuable time and I just can't believe this junk is required of everyone in the third year of medical school. Whoever designed this curriculum didn't know much about the education of a future radiologist. What I really need to know is how to read CT scans, interpret lab results, do a brief physical exam and then on to the real medicine. This other stuff is a waste of my time. It's much too touchy-feely. It may be fine for the weenies who want to go into Internal Medicine or Family Practice but we real doctors are men—and of course women—of action. At least my Advisor isn't one of those lightweights but a general surgeon who just might be able to understand that this course certainly isn't needed for us doctors who make things happen, but rather for those who are forever talking to patients. With this, the Student muttered under his breath, "Can we please get this show on the road?"

True to his word, in just a minute, the Advisor turned toward the Student, smiled and then raised the level of the lights in the room so that the room was fully lit. "Welcome to my home away from home," the Advisor said cheerfully.

"Thank you, sir," said the Student.

The Student looked at his Advisor for the first time and saw an almost bald, 60-ish man, with white hair in a circle around his head, glasses and a slight paunch. His face had somewhat of a hawkish nose with a kindly smile in place. He was wearing a dark blue golf shirt with an orange alligator on the pocket, a pair of khaki pants and some deck shoes without socks. *This is not how I expected a Professor of Surgery to dress. He must have come right off the golf course,* the Student thought.

This was the first meeting between the Student and his Advisor and was a requirement for all third-year medical students. Each needed to have an advisor who would guide them through the final two years of their medical school experience. The advisors played a powerful role in the medical students' lives, as they would help get various clerkships for the students, interface with the required clinical services and, most importantly, write the crucially important letter of recommendation to obtain a coveted residency. An advisor had the power to make or break a student at the medical school, so it was important to stay on his or her right side and to make the best impression possible.

The Student had asked many people about his Advisor but no one would say anything specific about him. They all made general, positive comments like, "He's a great guy. You'll love him," or "You're lucky. You'll learn a lot." When pushed for more specifics, they would all clam up or evade the question. The Student found this quite bizarre, as people in the medical school generally talked openly about anything except for politics and religion.

One resident finally told the Student under threat of bodily harm, "He's the best experience that I've ever had in my life. It's different for everyone so it's difficult to explain exactly what will happen to you. All that I can say is that you'll be challenged and stimulated like you've never been before in your life. There won't appear to be any rhyme or reason to what he does but then suddenly, one day, you'll realize how far you've come . . . and how much you've learned. I can't tell you more or it might ruin the experience for you." As he turned to leave, the resident laughed and mumbled, "You're going to go through some strange stuff before you leave that office." The Student didn't know what to think of this, since it was a psychiatry resident who made the comments and those people were known to be very strange anyway.

"Well, how do you like my office?" asked the Advisor.

Choosing his words carefully, the Student replied, "Well, Sir, it's a bit unusual. You don't sit behind the desk like all the other professors or doctors I've seen. Your desk is on the side against the wall and your computer is on the table in the back. There's nothing really separating us."

"Do you like that or would you prefer the more traditional layout?" asked the Advisor.

"Well, it's so different from what I've experienced before. Without the barrier of the desk, it's almost like sitting in a comfortable room at home rather than an office," said the Student.

"Precisely what I'd hoped for," smiled the Advisor. "Consider this your first lesson in the Art of Medicine. Anything that you can do to break down the barriers between the people you come in contact with or take care of is important. Communication between doctors and patients is difficult enough without having any artificial barriers between you. Creating the right environment is an important start to any communication process."

The Advisor leaned back and thought for a moment. "Do you remember how long it took to begin the peace negotiations to end the Vietnam War? What one of the biggest stumbling blocks to beginning the peace talks was?" he quizzed.

Good God, the Student thought. *The Vietnam War? Why is he going on about that? It was all but over before I was born. God, have I got myself a real winner for an advisor. We're going back to review ancient history. What has this got to do with patient care? What can I say that won't get him off on some other tangent?*

"No sir, I don't," answered the Student, trying not to show in his voice the irritation he felt.

"Well, it was the size and shape of the table they were going to sit around to work out the terms of a possible peace agreement. If the right atmosphere wasn't created in the beginning, if all parties to the process didn't feel like they were equal partners, then the process was doomed to fail. Something that we usually take as very insignificant held up the actual peace talks for months and cost countless lives on both sides. It seems ridiculous at one level, but does show how important the environment can be to achieving good communication," stated the Advisor.

"Well enough of that," he continued. "We'll deal more with barriers to good communication in the future. I know that you're getting ready to begin your clinical rotations next week so I thought it would be good for us to meet. Here's what we are going to do this week. I'd like it to serve as the general format for all our future meetings. I'm going to ask you to read something and then we'll have a discussion around that topic. When you begin seeing patients on your clinical rotations, I'll ask you to share some of those encounters with me so that we can discuss them as well. Questions?"

"Will we uh . . . will there be a quiz or test on this at the end?" the Student asked cautiously.

"No," laughed the Advisor. "What we discuss together won't be on any test I'll ever give but it will more likely be part of the evaluation done every day by every patient you see."

What is this guy thinking? the Student wondered. *How can the patients evaluate me? I'm going to be an interventional radiologist and really won't have to deal with many patients. And here*

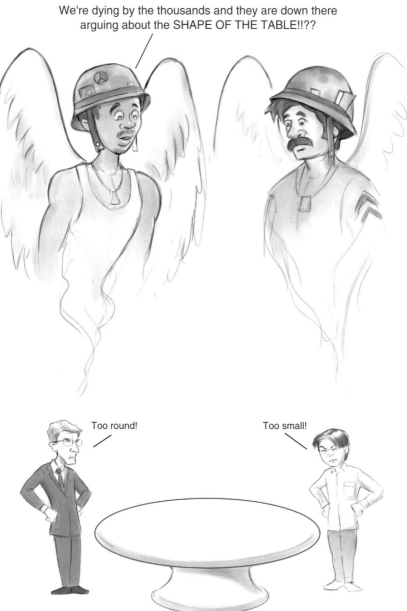

*in this med school, I don't think its even part of our evaluations.
This guy is one ham sandwich short of a picnic*, the Student
thought as he laughed to himself.

"O.K., then. Let's get started. I want you to go read this essay about what some doctors and patients are feeling today.
When you're finished reading it and you've thought about
it a bit, come back here and we'll discuss it together. I'll wait
around until you come back. Take as little or as long as you
want. Oh, there is one thing. I don't mind missing dinner
but I have tickets to the basketball game tonight and if I miss
that, I'll be really upset," the Advisor said, and the Student
thought he saw a twinkle in the older man's eye.

"Don't worry," the Student said as he took the essay. "I
can read pretty quickly, plus I'm not a big one for long discussions. See you in a few minutes."

True to his word, the Student returned within thirty minutes to the Advisor's office. He knocked and said, "Sorry to
interrupt but I've finished reading the article and I'm ready
to review it with you. I don't want to be the reason you miss
your game."

The Advisor laughed before replying, "I appreciate your
concern but don't worry about me so much. I'm more interested in getting to the heart of you. We've got a lot to
cover in these next couple of years if we're going to get you
ready for the real art of caring for people. So, what did you
think of the article I gave you on the changes taking place in
medicine?"

"Well, it was interesting but there have always been doctors and there have been patients so that's not going to
change."

The Advisor smiled before answering. "Student, let me
suggest to you that the changes affecting the practice of
medicine in recent years are some of the most dramatic in
the history of medicine. The paradigm for the doctor-
patient relationship may be forever changed because of

what's happened over the past several years. Here are the two things that I think have had—and will have—far ranging impacts on the future of medicine. The first is managed care and the second is easily accessible medical information, especially via the Internet and the television media. Do you have any idea why they've affected the doctor-patient relationship so much?"

"It's pretty easy to see how managed care has changed things so greatly because they pay for much of medical care today. It's the Golden Rule: 'He who has the gold makes the rules.' Managed care has set some new rules for how patients get care today but . . . but we've always had medical insurance companies."

"You're right. We've had medical insurance since the 1920s but never in the past have we ever had a layer of interference between the doctor and patient as we have today, and we have those wonderful folks in managed care to thank for all this. These MCOs, or managed care organizations, have basically destabilized the doctor-patient relationship by dictating where patients may go for medical care . . . and the saddest part is, it's all about money and rarely has anything to do with quality of care. Patients with long-standing relationships with their doctors are informed one day that their company has a new contract for medical benefits and their own doctor is no longer part of the covered services. So what happens? They have to see a new doctor and the relationship must be built from the beginning again. Neither patients nor physicians are in control. It's some corporate entity dictating how medicine is practiced."

The Advisor just shook his head sadly before continuing, "And that may only be the beginning. Physicians are forced in some situations to slash fees so that they are barely covering overhead. It doesn't even consider the increased paperwork, the rules and regulations like pre-certification review, the concern with 'cookbook medicine' and the overall emphasis on costs, and not quality. Medicare, for instance, pays only about half of a physician's usual fees, so those physicians can't even cover their office overhead. It's the primary reason that increasing numbers of physicians are refusing to see Medicare patients any longer and why Medicare MCOs are failing. What do physicians have to do then? They try to see more patients to make up for the loss of income brought about by sharply reduced fees. What do you think this does to the doctor-patient relationship?"

"It's got to cut down on the time physicians have to spend with their patients."

"Perfect! That's exactly what's happening and why both patients and physicians feel shortchanged and unhappy. To make any relationship work, it takes time and energy. These are two commodities most impacted by the need to see more people to make a reasonable income. Contrary to what you might read at times in the popular press, the motivation for almost all physicians—and for that matter other healthcare professionals—is NOT for the money but to help people. It's the primary reason cited in survey after survey. Sure, they get rewarded financially, but their biggest reward comes in the form of what I call 'emotional income'—the good feelings they get when their patients are happy and appreciative of the care they have been given. You might be having a really busy day with difficult problems to solve but at the end of the day you realize that you are energized—you feel great about the kind of job you did and the difference you made in the people you saw that day. It's when you are fully engaged in what you are doing that you get this 'emotional income.' And it's exactly this 'emotional income' that's been so severely compromised by managed care and the restraints put on physicians. This is probably the biggest reason why so many physicians are so unhappy today." The Student could see that his Advisor was obviously upset and agitated—and becoming increasingly animated.

"I can see I'm making you a bit nervous. Sorry, but it's hard for someone older like me to accept these changes because I feel that the bad clearly outweighs the good. I personally have seen patients with whom I've had a wonderful relationship for years have to leave because of changes in insurance. It gets me really, really irritated. Let me go on to point number two."

The Advisor got up and began to pace about the room. "The other very recent phenomenon that's changed the whole world and the way we communicate that's also had a significant impact on medicine has been the Internet. Because of all the information that is readily accessible to the average person on the Internet today, it has forever changed the balance of power between doctor and patient. For the <u>first time</u> in the history of medicine, a patient, a consumer of medical services, can, with some effort, attain an amount of medical knowledge that is equal to or greater than a physician when it comes to certain specific illnesses within medicine. In the past, patients didn't really have easy access to a vast amount of medical information. Now, you can learn to do heart surgery or make some obscure medical diagnosis using the information found on the Internet. The dynamics of the doctor-patient relationship have been changed forever."

"Is that a bad thing?" the Student asked somewhat timidly.

"No, definitely not, but what it does do is drastically change the rules and protocols by which patients and doctors have interacted for centuries. Doctors no longer have a monopoly on medical knowledge so now the patient can challenge, ask questions and frankly, become an equal when it comes to certain esoteric diseases. What's causing so much chaos and unhappiness in medical practices all over the country today is the stress created by the changes in the doctor-patient dynamic. Both the patient and the doctor have learned the old rules of interacting from parents, from how things are depicted on television, and from our own personal experiences, but the paradigm is changing dramatically—and no one has done a good job of defining the new rules and protocols for how doctors and patients can work together so that each gets what they want out of the healing relationship."

The Advisor sat back down and then spoke earnestly to his student, "Part of what I see us working on together over your final two years is helping you develop the tools to enable you and your patients to cope successfully with all the changes in medicine. I'd also like to identify what your dreams are, what you think will make you happy in life, and help you attain it." He stopped then and looked closely at the Student. "Do you know how to eat an elephant?"

The Student looked like the proverbial deer caught in the headlights. *Is this a trick question? Where is this guy coming from? Maybe it's not too late to change advisors. Please just get me out of here.*

The Advisor chuckled before replying; "I see I surprised you with that question. You eat an elephant one bite at a time. You learn about medicine and yourself in the same way. You don't learn all of what we were talking about overnight. It takes time to think about it and to process it. Any profession takes time to master. I heard Harrison Ford, the actor, say in an interview on Bravo the other night that he felt acting was like building a brick wall. You build it brick by brick, one layer at a time. It's the same way you learn any craft or profession. It's the same for a mechanic, a builder, a lawyer or an athlete. Medicine is no different. It takes time to learn the Art and Science of Medicine. I know I hit you with a lot in this first meeting but I hope it will all make sense to you down the road. Now, any questions for me before we finish our first session?"

"Well, as a matter of fact, yes," said the Student. "When I first knocked on the door today and you had your back to me, how did you know it was me at the door and that I was wearing a tie?"

"Do you really want to know the answer?" grinned the Advisor.

"Yeah," he said with a pause. " I would."

"Well, it's actually fairly elementary . . . a very simple bit of deductive reasoning. I knew that it was time for our appointment and your knock on the door sounded tentative at best so I guessed it was you. As for the second part of your question, I know from past experience that almost all the male medical students wear ties to impress faculty in the beginning, and especially when they visit the head of general surgery. I played the odds and this time, the house won. Now, get out of here," he said with a laugh.

✤ *Perspectives for Doctors* ✤

Physicians are angry, frustrated and not getting what they want from their patients

Patients are also angry, frustrated and not getting what they want from their doctors.

In a recent article, one of the most prestigious national medical journals, *The New England Journal of Medicine,* stated, "Many American doctors are unhappy with the quality of their professional lives." How bad is it? Many physicians are now looking at other career opportunities outside of the active practice of medicine. A *New York* magazine article, and articles in a number of regional newspapers over the past year, has served to further highlight this problem.

What's going on? How can both groups be experiencing the same emotions and inner turmoil? How can both not be getting their needs met from the way medicine is being practiced today? Is there a solution that's a "win-win" for both doctors and patients? I believe there is, and that solution is what this book is all about.

In my job as a national medical reporter for NBC News, I've had the opportunity to speak to hundreds of doctors about their careers in medicine. One question I always ask is, "Would you encourage your children to undertake a career in medicine?" With rare exception, most physicians answer that question a very strong "No." My next question was always, "Why?"

Their answers were all basically the same, in that they all mention one or all of the following issues: 1) managed care companies put so many limits on the time I can spend with patients; 2) so many groups are second-guessing what I do after the fact; 3) all employers and insurance companies care about is saving money and not the quality of care delivered; 4) I feel like I don't have enough time for my patients anymore; and 5) I feel like I'm always practicing defensive medicine just to avoid some ridiculous lawsuit.

What about the patient side of the equation? Why are they so frustrated and angry? Doctors need to know why so we can help work toward solutions that will make the lives of both patients and doctors better. My job at NBC has also allowed me the opportunity to speak to and interview many patients. One thing has become obvious: Patients would tell me things that they had never told their physicians. Why? They said they were afraid to upset their doctors or felt it wouldn't do any good. A recent study confirms this very fact. Eighty-five percent of patients leave physician practices without providing an explanation, and they leave at a rate of about fifteen percent per year. How can physicians possibly be expected to change if they don't even know what the problem is? None of us would want to be treated in that manner, especially in relationships that were important to us.

In addition, my twenty-three years working as an ER physician have provided me a great forum for finding out what concerns patients. It should be no surprise that patients care about many of the same issues. The number one concern of patients . . . **Doctors just don't seem to have enough time for them.** In too many cases, the perception of the medical-care consumer, the patient, is that doctors breeze in and breeze out of exam rooms with only a brief encounter with the patient. Instead, the people spending the most time with patients seem to be the support staff or physician extenders such as nurse practitioners or physician assistants. Managed care companies add to the problem by denying services or making it difficult to access healthcare. In the interest of cost saving, companies are cutting back on the amount of services provided under their medical benefits plans, or they are forcing employees to pay more for the same services. All of these factors contribute to the terrible frustration and subsequent anger that patients feel today and, in many cases, transfer to us as doctors.

Many medical schools do have some type of course or introduction to the Art of Medicine but the content and the length of these offerings vary greatly from school to school. Often, they are short courses and viewed as a necessary evil by students before getting to the real meat of their studies, the clinical rotations. In many cases, it's an attempt by schools to pay some half-hearted homage to "bedside manner" without really meaning it, and this is exactly where the problem lies.

If you think back to how we learned, even from our earliest days as toddlers, it was by repetition. Each task we learned by doing over and over again. We all got sick of saying our "times tables" again and again, or maybe it was conjugating verbs in a foreign language repeatedly, but that's what it took to ingrain things into our memories. Only in this way does information become comfortable for us. Trust me, the same kind of learning takes place in medical schools all over the country. The things that are important are repeated over and over again until they become second nature to students or residents. One of the problems in learning the Art of Medicine and all the skills that go along with it is that the necessary skills are not constantly stressed or repeated. The emphasis instead is on the Science of Medicine. If medical schools don't constantly reinforce the importance of the "bedside manner," then it won't become a habit. It won't become something that's comfortable for students.

One of the major problems with medical students, residents and young doctors is that many of them are emotionally immature and naïve about life in the "real" world. That's a pretty damning statement but until they go into practice, many of them live in a very isolated and somewhat protective environment. One of the weaknesses of the medical educational system is that most medical students go from high school to college to medical school directly. Students enter medical school at age twenty-one or twenty-two. They rarely experience life outside of the protective environment provided by the U.S. educational system except for that part of their lives "lived" in their individual family, social class, or community. The majority of medical students don't understand what it's like to have a job that's the primary source of income for a family. They don't understand that if a wage earner doesn't work, the family may not have food, clothing or housing. Most have been protected from all this. It's not in their realm of experience. All that most have had to do is focus on learning science and facts.

When students move to their clinical years and start learning how to take care of patients, they learn from those above them in their training, as well as faculty and other healthcare professionals. Unless certain behaviors are modeled and expected of them, then they won't learn these behaviors, nor will they be willing to incorporate them into the way they deal with patients. In some ways it's just like parenting. If you don't have good role models that expect and demand certain ways of treating and respecting people, then your chances of doing so are considerably less.

Many medical schools do have advisors for medical students but rarely do they really follow students as they go through their clinical years. This is almost always left to faculty who happen to be teaching on a particular clinical rotation. Generally, students learn from observing how faculty and residents deal with patients. It is extremely rare to get the personal attention paid by the Advisor in this chapter, but it certainly would make a difference in what students would perceive as being important. Like anything else in life, it can be inferred that where people put their time and energy is where their priorities lie. You can say that you value your family life above all other things but if you don't devote much time and energy to your family, then you're not walking the walk. Likewise, medical schools may say that the Art of Medicine is important but if they don't devote sufficient time to it, or evaluate students on how well they model its components, and then it's only so much lip service. You've got to put your money where your mouth is.

Dr. Stephen Covey wrote a best-selling book titled *The 7 Habits of Highly Effective People.* In that book, Covey makes the point that one of the things that highly successful people do so well is to set very specific goals and then work toward them. Without goals, you are like a rudderless ship; the tide can take you anywhere. No business would be successful without specific, well-defined goals that are communicated to everyone in the organization. If you didn't have certain expectations or goals for your children, then they could do whatever they wanted. It just doesn't work. Without goals, you are doomed to failure and everyone will soon be unhappy. Keep in mind the old saying, "If you keep on doing what you're doing, then you're going to keep on getting what you're getting." This is why one of Dr. Covey's key first principles is "Begin with the end in mind."

During my years in the emergency room, there was nothing more frustrating than to see a patient with a rambling story and a variety of complaints. My biggest problem was trying to figure out why he or she really came to the ER. I always believed that for most people to come to the ER to be seen, something had changed or was bothering them enough to make a difference in their life. My job was to figure out what that was. I always wished that these patients had thought out what their real goal was for that ER visit. It would have made them a lot happier and saved me a lot of time, tests and heartburn.

It Takes Two to Tango . . . and Communicate

The Student and the Advisor had agreed to meet at 9:45 a.m. in the Lown Patient Educational Center. The Center was named for Dr. Bernard Lown, a world-famous cardiologist and the author of a renowned book on the Art of Healing. It was to be the Student's first experience with a standardized patient. The use of standardized patients was becoming more common in many medical schools. These "patients" were not really sick but were ordinary people drawn from the local community, and they were trained to simulate a particular medical problem for medical students and residents. Often, these patients might be actors, people who'd had a particular disease in the past, or more commonly, just everyday people who wanted to help doctors in training develop patient interviewing skills.

The Lown Patient Educational Center comprised many large examination rooms, all equipped with cameras and audio equipment, so that each patient interview could be videotaped in a central control room. There were also smaller rooms in which the teachers could review the tapes with the students and the standardized patients. There were study carrels for students and residents; these had computers that could access the Internet and run the latest CD-ROM educational programs. All this high-tech gear had one primary purpose—to enhance the young doctors'-in-training communication skills with patients.

The Advisor came into the Center shortly after the Student, and immediately noticed his advisee sitting in a corner chair of the waiting room. He had a book in his hand but was staring into space while his foot tapped nervously up and down on the floor.

"Hello there, Student, how's it going today? You a little nervous about your first videotape session with one of our standardized patients?"

"No, Sir, why do you say that?" asked the Student but with no real conviction in his voice.

"Oh, no special reason, but maybe it has something to do with your body language—the foot tapping, squirming in your seat and staring into space that I observed when I came in. As my mom used to say, 'You look like you're sitting on pins and needles.' You know, it's O.K. to be nervous and I'd be surprised if you weren't. Anytime any of us do something new, it's potentially stressful but with careful preparation, including rehearsal, you can reduce your anxiety considerably. That's why I'm here . . . to help you learn the Art of Medicine and to make you successful."

"Can you really make this whole patient thing easier? One of the reasons I want to go into radiology is because I want something I can measure and quantify. I like talking to my friends but I don't want to waste a lot of time talking to people I don't know. I'm not one who has a need to have long-term relationships with the people I see. This interviewing stuff is for those touchy-feely types in my class. I personally don't see the need for it all."

The Advisor nodded his head, sighed and said, "I hear what you're saying but let me try and give you a little different perspective on this. Let's imagine for a moment that you're a radiologist and that you've been asked by another physician to perform a particular test like an MRI on a patient. You have a couple of options. You can perform the test as ordered, or by actually speaking to the patient and listening to his complaints, you discover that another, more focused radiologic test would be better at getting to the bottom of the patient's complaints. By taking a history, by talking to the patient, you have not only saved the patient time and money but also done away with unnecessary testing that fails to elucidate his or her problem. This is why you need to learn how to speak to patients. Make sense?"

"Yeah, when you put it that way, it sure does. I still don't like it but it could have some usefulness in the long run . . . maybe."

"All right, you've got two years of clinical rotations to do and lots of patients to examine so let me give you some tips that should make it easier for you. First, you only have one chance to make a first impression so give it your best shot from the very beginning. You can do some simple things from the get-go that will help improve the doctor-patient relationship. It starts from the moment you enter the exam room. Walk in with a smile, shake the patient's hand and introduce yourself. These are all simple courtesies but it's amazing how often they're neglected. They set the tone for your relationship with the patient immediately."

They walked back toward the exam room where the Student's standardized patient was waiting for him. The Advisor continued, "One thing that you're sure to see when examining patients with other doctors—and that I NEVER want to see you do with any patient—is to walk in the room while looking at the chart and begin talking to the patient without looking at him or her. Why do you think I feel so strongly about this one point?"

"Um . . . is it because they have more experience than I do and can get away with it?"

"No, it has nothing at all to do with experience. It has a great deal to do with communication with your patient. Every person communicates with another person in three ways—by what they say; by their body language; and by how they say it, their paralanguage. If you're not looking at the patient, you will miss two of the three ways that a patient is communicating with you. Here's a good rule to remember. If there's a discrepancy between the words that are being said and the body language, then believe the body language. If you're looking at the chart and not the patient, you will miss a great deal of what the patient is really trying to tell you . . . or trying to hide from you. Now get in there and have fun. I'll be back after my meeting with the dean to see how it went for you."

Have fun? Is he kidding me? I'm scared to death. At least this person isn't really sick so I'm not likely to cause any harm but I hate that I'm being watched. I wish they'd turn that damn videotape off. I know how to talk to people. Why do I need this stuff? What a waste of time? Oh well, here goes nothing!

With that the Student entered the room with the patient and his session began. In about fifteen minutes the Student returned to the reviewing room. Dr. Robert Watson, the head of the Center, would be reviewing the tape with the Student, along with the standardized patient. They all sat down in front of the tape machine and watched the entire encounter before anyone spoke. Dr. Watson began the session.

"Well, Student, how did you think it went with your patient?"

The Student smiled before replying, "I thought it went well. My patient complained of some tingling in her fingers when she moved her body in certain ways. I asked some questions, did my exam and came to what I thought was a likely diagnosis. I even suggested some testing that would help make a definitive diagnosis."

"Do you think that your patient, Mrs. Cullen, was pleased with your encounter?"

"I would hope so. I made the likely diagnosis so I can't imagine what more she'd want."

Dr. Watson then turned to the patient, Mrs. Cullen. "How did you think your meeting went?"

Mrs. Cullen turned and faced the Student before replying, "I was pleased with the initial impression you made. You greeted me with a smile and a handshake as well as your name. You then asked my reason for coming to see you today. You asked some questions around my complaint that were appropriate and then you proceeded directly to the hands-on physical examination. You then told me that I needed to have some testing and you'd set it up for me. You then told me—as you were leaving with your hand on the door—that I needed to avoid using my wrist for the next two weeks. You'd then see me back after that time and when the results were in. Did I fairly characterize our encounter, Student?" asked Mrs. Cullen.

"Yes, that seems right," the Student replied happily.

Mrs. Cullen continued at this point, "Let's look at the tape now together and let me point out a few things as we watch it."

The tape began to play from the point when the Student entered the room.

"One of the things that I did not like, and can be seen here, is that the Student remained standing during his history taking. It gave me the feeling that he was in a hurry and made me feel somewhat uncomfortable. I always prefer my doctor to sit down so that it seems like he or she is talking with me the way a friend might. The other thing that you'll notice is how you'd ask me a question, then you'd be looking at the chart and writing as I'd answer it. You couldn't possibly see the reaction on my face or my body language in some cases. I actually put in some gestures to prove my point. See, here I'm sticking out my tongue at you and then wagging my finger like I'm scolding you as you write. You had no idea I was doing it."

At that point, the Student turned visibly red.

Dr. Watson spoke up at that point. "I know you're feeling a bit embarrassed at this point but that's the reason we do this now before you start seeing patients. You're in no way unusual in what you did with Mrs. Cullen. As you make rounds in the hospital, I'm sure that you're going to see many physicians who will write in or read charts while patients are talking to them. It's a bad habit that many physicians have and that they're not even aware is a problem. It may be that it's never been pointed out to them but since you know about it now, you can consciously avoid this *faux pas* as you see patients. What else, Mrs. Cullen?"

"As you know, I've been a standardized patient for several years now and I've seen hundreds of students and physicians. One common problem that they all have is an excessive focus on the chief complaint to the almost total exclusion of the rest of me. How can you adequately treat me if you don't know me in the context of the rest of my life? For example, when you were taking my history, you never asked me how this problem affected me in my daily activities of living or on my job. If you had, I would have given you many examples of the impact of my wrist problem on my daily life. I can't lift my young children without pain. I can't type for long periods on my job without feeling increased tingling. I wake up at night with pain that affects my lifestyle in many ways.

"Another question that I hoped you would ask, but you didn't, and that I think every patient would like to be asked, is what I thought the problem might be and what I did on a daily basis to make it worse or better. This would provide you some real insights on how to treat the problem, and then you might focus some of your answers or proposed testing to help address my concerns. Do you agree with that, Dr. Watson?"

"Yes, I do. Great points. Let's stop the tape for a minute." With that he leaned over and pushed the pause button on the VCR machine.

"For the most part, patients come to us because something is bothering them enough to impact their life in a negative way. They want it fixed. Remember, the chief complaint is only that—a chief complaint. It's a place to start but it may not have any relationship to the real underlying problem that is the cause of a patient's distress." Dr. Watson paused and turned back to the Student.

"Let me give you a real life example. I had a twenty-three-year-old woman come to me complaining of abdominal pain. She had been to several doctors who did numerous tests including endoscopy, a GI series, and CT scans. All were negative. Various medicines were tried without success. She was referred to me for another opinion. I reviewed all the previous studies for myself as one should never trust someone else's opinion, since it might not be as described and you do the patient a real disservice.

"I then took a social history of the patient and found that she still lived at home with her parents. She had been engaged for several months to a young man about whom her parents had fairly negative feelings. She too had very unsure feelings about her fiancé but didn't want to appear to be caving in to her parents. She had always been the type of person who worked at pleasing everyone. This obviously set up a scenario for her that caused tremendous conflict and one in which she would end up hurting someone. As the date for her wedding drew closer and the planning started, her stomach problems worsened. Not one of her other physicians had taken a real social history. It's no wonder that all her costly, invasive tests came back as negative or normal. It takes more effort and definitely more time but it's what makes the difference between a good physician and a great one."

At that point, his Advisor came back into the conference room. "How's it going?" he asked pleasantly.

Dr. Watson got up and greeted him warmly, "Glad you could join us again. We're almost done here. Anything else, Mrs. Cullen?"

"Why don't you let the tape play to the end? I've got just a couple more points that I noted. When you discussed testing, you didn't really give me any options or ask me if that was acceptable to me. If you had, you might have learned that I was pregnant and that a CT scan was probably something to be avoided if possible."

The Student noticeably reddened again and squirmed uneasily in his seat.

Damn, how could I make such a dumb mistake? Anybody knows that you have to think about every woman of childbearing age being pregnant. This woman must think I'm the stupidest medical student she's ever had. What a time for my Advisor to come in! My first real experience with a patient and I blow it right in front of him.

As if she were reading his thoughts, Mrs. Cullen continued. "Don't think you're the only one making that same

I see on your chart that we had you on fertility drugs a couple years ago.

Any luck with that?

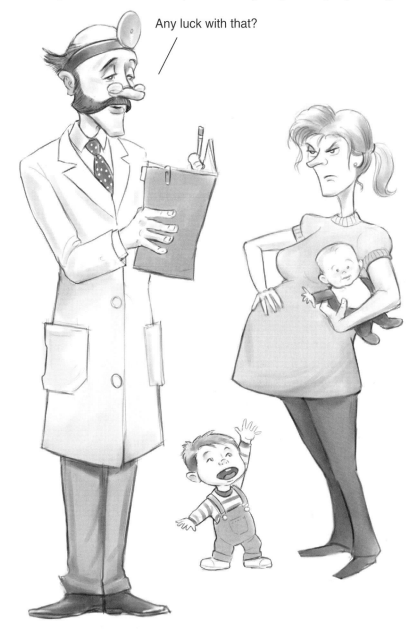

mistake, Student. Almost every medical student and resident who has examined me has failed to ask me whether or not I was pregnant. It's a great lesson to learn now and not one you'd like to learn on a real patient."

She looked at the Student for a moment before continuing, "Another bit of advice that I have to offer you relates to the way you exited the room. You moved to the door like you were in a hurry to leave and had somewhere to go. Then, you told me not to use my wrist for two weeks. That would be impossible for me to do because I have small children at home. You didn't know that since you never asked if I had any problems with your instructions. I'd suggest you always check with a patient to see if they have any problems complying with a treatment regimen. You'll learn a great deal that way."

The Advisor laughed at that point. "It reminds me of when I was an intern on surgery. One of the duties that interns got then was writing prescriptions for patients when they left the hospital after surgery. I had just written a prescription for this one patient and handed it to him, telling him to get it filled and start taking it right away. He then told me that he had no money, since he'd lost his job because of his chronic surgical problem. What I did wrong was that I failed to ask the patient if there would be any problems or barriers with him complying with our treatment plan. It's a basic mistake that many physicians forget to consider. I have to remind my residents all the time about this very issue. You'll learn so much about your patient and his or her life when you ask that simple question before leaving a patient."

Dr. Watson chimed in at that point. "You have to be very direct with patients when you communicate. Leave no room for error. Ask them directly, 'Is there anything you know of that will prevent you from following the treatment plan that we've just gone over together? Are there any barriers to your getting and taking the medicine I've pre-scribed?' You have to be that direct. Trust me.

"You also have to be very direct in the instructions you give regarding medicines. For instance, I had one lady who failed to take off the aluminum foil wrapper before insert-ing the rectal suppository I'd prescribed. It seemed obvious to me but now I give each patient that specific instruction in a light-hearted way." With that the whole group laughed and the slight tension in the room was eased.

Mrs. Cullen again turned to the Student and continued, "The final point that I'd like to make is that you never asked me if I understood what you said to me. You also never asked me if I had any questions. It's always extremely com-forting when my personal physician asks me if I have any questions or issues that she hasn't yet addressed. I believe that it's a wonderful way of demonstrating her care and concern for me. As someone on the receiving end of your care, I'd strongly suggest that you add this to the list of things you do for each of your patients before ending any encounter. Do you doctors agree?"

"Absolutely," the Advisor said with great enthusiasm. "If you assume that the patient understands or hears every-thing you say, then you've done a disservice to him or her. When you 'assume,' you make an 'ass' out of 'u' and 'me.'

"Mrs. Cullen, thanks for your help. You've helped to give a great many of our students the proper start in the Art of Medicine. Now, I'm going to give my Student a little article to read that may reinforce some of the points you've made today."

Mrs. Cullen and Dr. Watson left the room but the Advisor stayed while the Student read the article. He waited to speak until after the Student was done reading.

"Did you feel kind of stupid today when we reviewed the videotape with you and pointed out some of the things that needed improvement?"

"Yeah, I sure did. Some of the things that I failed to do were so blatant. I couldn't believe that I did so badly. I always thought that I communicated well with people."

With that comment, the Advisor just chuckled. "I'm not laughing at you and, believe it or not, you didn't do that badly. You play basketball, don't you?"

The Student nodded but clearly looked puzzled.

"The reason I asked that question is to try and relate to you in terms that you'll easily understand. It's something that you'll find extremely helpful when dealing with any patient you'll see in the future as well.

"When you first began playing basketball, you probably weren't very good. You missed more shots than you made, dribbling the ball was awkward at best, and even making a simple lay-up was difficult. But what happened when you stuck to it and you got some coaching from your father or a coach at school? With time and practice, you got better and better and better. All skills and all sports are learned behaviors. You improve over time but it takes practice, repetition, and some coaching or instruction. Taking a medical history and communicating with patients are absolutely no different. You learn by doing and, like most of us, you learn your most unforgettable lessons by your own or others' mistakes. I wish that weren't so but it's just the way life is. Now, what's the ONE other thing that each person must have in order to get better at whatever he's trying to do?"

The Student frowned, thought for a minute and just shook his head, " I'm not sure."

"Desire," the Advisor exclaimed with a smile. "If you don't want to improve, if you don't have that fire inside you to get better at whatever you're doing, then no amount of coaching will make a difference. There's no substitute for hard work . . . it takes time and effort at practice to see improvement. At the same time, if you practice the wrong things, then you won't get better either. That's why you need a good coach. Frankly, medicine is no different. You need good physicians as your role models or teachers to help you work on the right things."

At that point, Dr. Watson came back into the room after he had finished thanking Mrs. Cullen and reviewing her schedule for the next week. It was always busier when the new students and residents began their medical rotations.

"Bob, we were just talking about the need for role models in medicine. Was that helpful for you when you were learning how to take care of patients?"

"You better believe it. There are very few physicians who are naturals and possess all the skills required to totally care for their patients. There are very few Michael Jordan's of medicine. Some may be very good at history taking but lack basic skills in communication, listening or performing a physical exam. We all need role models or physicians who teach by their example. Sir William Osler is often cited as one of those who served as a role model for so many doctors. Dr. Bernard Lown, the man for whom this center is named, wrote a book titled *The Lost Art of Healing*. In it, Dr. Lown recalls how he spent years learning the Art of Medicine by watching and listening to Dr. Peter Levine, his Chief of Cardiology. He provides many examples of what his great teacher did at the bedside to show him how to take care of those entrusted to them."

The Advisor chimed in at that point, "One of the problems we have in medicine today is that there are so few doctors who can serve as good role models. The really good ones are often overrun with patients and their time is short due to all their other responsibilities. You've got to understand that physicians are not reimbursed by insurance carriers for the quality of their care, and the manner in which we reward medical school faculty rarely considers superior teaching or the excellence of their patient care. It's a sad commentary on our times," he said with obvious regret.

With that, the Advisor sighed, got slowly out of his chair and headed for the door. "Let's go, Student. We've bent your ear enough for today. You need to get out of here. Just think about what you've seen and heard today. Remember, none of the coursework that you've taken to date or your limited life experiences has prepared you in any way for your interactions with patients. These are new skills that take time to learn, just like anatomy, biochemistry, and the other basic sciences. They all build on one another. Don't be discouraged. Believe it or not, you did well for your first time. There's one thing I can promise you: It's only going to get better."

It's so overwhelming. It's all so new and there's so much to learn. I do like the old guy's analogy to basketball. It makes so much sense. I wasn't very good at first but with practice I did become pretty damn good, if I say so myself.

The Student smiled and thanked everyone for his or her time. They got back to the front door of the Lown Center and headed off in different directions. The day was going to be another long for them all, and full of many challenges.

❖ *Perspectives for Doctors* ❖

All interactions between a doctor or healthcare professional and a patient begin with an initial encounter. It can be a single encounter never to be repeated again, such as when a patient is seen in the emergency room for some acute problem, is treated, and then sent to another physician for follow-up care if needed. The initial meeting could also be the first of many encounters that ultimately lead to a relationship that extends over time. Regardless, there is always an initial meeting, a coming together of two people for the first time with each person bringing his or her own needs, past experiences, expectations and desired outcomes to that encounter. Another way of thinking about this initial meeting is that it's almost like a first date.

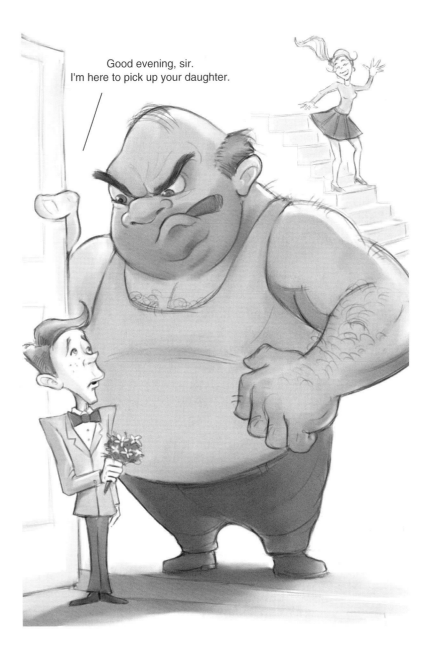

Think back to any first date you've had in the past. You're a little (or in my case a lot) nervous because you're not sure of how it's going to unfold or how you're likely to get along. You each bring certain expectations to the date. Where will it lead? How successful it will be? All of your past experiences with similar first-date situations will influence how you will think about this date. Will I get another date? Will he or she like me? Is this person likely to be one with whom I'll have a long-term relationship? Even if your paths may never cross again, the impact that first date, that single meeting, has on your psyche can be profound.

The first encounter between a physician and a patient can also be profound and have an impact that can last for years into the future, especially if it occurs in a young person or is associated with some strong emotional event, such as learning you have cancer or a serious disease. Don't think that the impact of an encounter affects only patients. These same feelings, reactions and emotions take place in all doctors as well. Unfortunately, with time, many doctors become less affected by these meetings with patients. As a defense mechanism, they learn to depersonalize these meetings and focus instead on the disease or illness, as the surgeon did in the introduction.

First meetings are so important. Remember the old saying? *"You only have one chance to make a first impression."* First impressions are key to any relationship and are extremely difficult to change. The interaction that takes place in that first meeting between doctor and patient (like the first date) often determines the course of future interactions between people. Was there a positive chemistry between the parties? Did the patient and/or the doctor have their needs met? Was the overall experience positive or negative? Did the patient feel good about the kind of care he received? Did the doctor think he did a good job and that his skills and talent were appreciated? How all these questions are answered can affect the course of future encounters between doctor and patient.

In many cases, first encounters lead to many more visits with a doctor or healthcare professional. What occurs in subsequent meetings can also affect the relationship but often with numerous meetings, the chance for positive experiences improves greatly. In future chapters, we'll learn how relationships evolve and what it takes to keep them going at a certain level so that they are stress-free and nurturing.

As is the case in the introduction, one of the most important factors in how a patient perceives a meeting with the doctor depends on his or her experiences with the doctor's office personnel. The first impression that a patient has of a doctor's practice takes place with the front office staff and the nursing personnel. Just think back to both positive and negative contacts you've had with office personnel and then how that affected your mood with the doctor.

Over the twenty-three years I spent working in the ER, I became extremely adept at quickly sensing a patient's mood when I walked into the room to see him or her for the first time. It was especially easy to sense, from both verbal and non-verbal communications, when he or she was upset or angry. I also learned that the best course of action was to immediately confront the situation and ask what was wrong or what was upsetting him or her so much. The most common reason for anger was the rudeness or disrespect a nurse or support person had shown while in the ER. The other thing that made patients really angry was the amount of time they spent in the waiting room prior to being examined. They could never understand why some patients were seen right away or why it took so long to be seen when the ER might not have seemed especially busy. I had to spend more time than I ever wanted just trying to defuse that situation before the healing encounter could begin. Fortunately, good support staff is more often the rule rather than the exception.

Smart physicians and intelligent hospital administrators have learned that hiring staff with strong communication and people skills is perhaps the single most important thing that they can do to improve the healing relationship.

Insensitive communication, poor communication, or a lack of communication as demonstrated above seems to be at the heart of the majority of problems between physicians and their patients. We all know horror stories about doctors who have been rude, cold, callous or just insensitive. We also know anecdotes about doctors who are at the opposite end of the spectrum. They are kind, sensitive, caring, seem to have time for patients and listen to what patients are trying to say. It is this latter approach that is at the heart of the Art of Medicine. **How good or bad a doctor is at the Art of Medicine is the single biggest factor affecting a patient's perception of his or her doctor and the root cause of a great many malpractice suits.**

Helping the sick means more than just treating their symptoms; it means offering them humor, compassion and friendship. It means treating them as real people with the total range of emotional needs. To do this it takes knowing the person you are caring for, and it's only by putting time and energy into communicating with a person that a trusting relationship gets built.

Why are family physicians sued so rarely compared to the surgical specialists? Most often it's because family practice doctors establish a relationship with their patients. They come to know their patients over a number of visits through sickness and health, through the good and bad. (Yes, it is like a marriage in some ways.) Many a patient has been heard to say that they know that old Dr. So-and-So may not have done everything right, and maybe even done a number of things wrong, "but we've known him or her for years and he's like part of our family. He did the best he could." A relationship has been established rather than an impersonal, isolated, cold encounter.

A physician may have a tremendous grasp of the technical or scientific aspects of medicine but if he or she lacks the communication skills needed to relate to the patient all those best efforts may be for naught—"the surgery was a success but unfortunately, the patient died."

Communication implies a dialogue or exchange of information between two people. In previous times, the doctor-patient relationship was often a monologue. The doctor, healthcare professional or hospital set the rules with little or no input from those receiving the service. The best physicians, those skilled in the Art of Medicine, quickly understood the need for listening to the stories that people want and need to tell if patients are to be served at the highest possible level.

The best medicine requires a dialogue. It requires two people interacting as partners to maximize the physician-patient relationship. A partnership implies responsibilities on both sides of the relationship. In many cases, patients have not understood nor accepted their responsibilities in this regard. Further chapters in this book will provide specific steps or techniques for both the physician and the patient, devised to help each learn what they can do to improve the physician-patient relationship and maximize the healing process. Only then will the Art of Medicine be valued and flourish as an integral part of the healing relationship.

Many medical schools do in fact use standardized patients as a way of training medical students and residents. There is much debate within the medical community as to the ultimate impact of these standardized patients on a person's ability to learn the Art of Medicine. I have to believe that if you are never exposed to the proper way to approach patients, then you might never know what the ideal should be.

In medicine, you can never diagnose a disease if you've never heard of or learned about that disease. Medical students or residents most frequently learn about a disease by reading about the "idealized" presentation or version of it in a textbook. For instance, students learn that patients with diabetes urinate frequently (polyuria), are always thirsty (polydypsia), eat frequently (polyphagia) and have weight loss. This often is not the way "real" patients communicate their symptoms to the doctor. Many a medical student has been known to lament, "The patient obviously hasn't read the book." What nerve! The advantage of listening to a standardized patient tell her story is to help the student learn how to draw out the story of a particular disease while understanding that not all the "ideal" elements of a disease need to be present for that disease to be present. Diabetics may only have one or may have all of the symptoms often associated with the disease.

Students or residents also learn about particular diseases from lectures, or in Grand Rounds or morbidity and mortality conferences. The final way of learning how diseases appear—or "present"—in individual patients is by interviewing patients with a particular medical problem. Because each of us is so wonderfully unique due to our individual genetic makeup, the way a particular disease affects us can also be just as unique. It is up to the practitioner to listen to the story the patient tells, and to make sense out of it. It's only by learning good communication skills and appropriate techniques that we maximize the chances of extracting the real story from our patients.

Listening—the Key to Healing

"Listening, not imitation, is the sincerest form of flattery. Listening is unspoken caring."

–Sir William Osler

"Be a good listener because you never learn much from talking."

–Will Rogers

It was the first of July and the appointed day for all the new residents in the hospital and all third-year medical students to begin the first day on their respective medical rotations. The common wisdom in medical circles was that you'd better not get sick around July 1st because nothing good was likely to happen due to the arrival of all these new, inexperienced doctors and students. In fact, many nurses tried to take their vacations then because they hated dealing with these new arrivals, fresh out of medical school, who were often afraid to admit their ignorance or ask for help from anyone who was not a doctor.

The Emergency Medicine service was no exception to this rule. The twelve first-year residents in Emergency Medicine and the twenty-four students beginning their ER rotations were all gathered together to hear a lecture on caring for patients, given by one of the attending physicians. The nervousness among the group was almost palpable as they waited. They were eager to get going but so afraid to actually begin seeing patients. The little chatter that took place in the packed conference room was all small talk. No one knew what to expect from his or her first day on the rotation.

The door opened and in walked the attending physician. He had a slide carousel under his arm and was carrying a large, black exercise bag. He was tall, looked to be in his early sixties and had a few extra pounds on his frame. "Good morning," he said. "I'm sure you're all feeling a bit nervous and anxious to get going. I know I sure was when I was a new resident. My chief resident then was a good old boy from Alabama—and he knew, and used, every old Southern aphorism that you could ever imagine. One of his favorites that comes to mind when looking at all of you today is 'You all are as nervous as a long-tailed cat in a room full of rocking chairs.' There were a few other things he used to say but I can't repeat them as I'd definitely be in trouble with the dean."

The group exploded with nervous laughter and everyone relaxed a bit.

"I'm Dr. Peter Rosen, this month's attending in Emergency Medicine. I asked for my vacation these next two weeks so that I wouldn't have to deal with any of you but I obviously drew the short straw in the department." He stopped at that point to survey the room and was again met by all smiles.

"Hey, loosen up, ladies and gentleman! You're all as serious as a heart attack. You're going to need a sense of humor as you go through your training. If you don't find one soon, it's going to be a long three years for you here in the ER." With that he smiled and pulled from his bag a multicolored hat with a blue propeller on top. He put it on his head and then pulled a large red clown's nose out as well and placed that on his nose. The sight was extremely comical and most again chuckled but a few had unsure expressions on their faces.

"I can see from the expressions on some of your faces that you're thinking I'm a little strange. If you should ever talk to my wife and kids, they'd definitely confirm that opinion for you but that's not why I'm wearing this. These are some of the things in my bag of ER tricks that I use as icebreakers for some of our young patients. When they see me in some of these things, they immediately begin to loosen up and they forget why they're in the ER and that they're scared out of their wits. It's only when they finally relax a bit that they'll usually begin talking to me. When I let them actually wear some of this stuff, they're all mine, and they'll really listen to what I'm saying to them. I've got their attention and they've got mine, and that's what it takes with all of our patients here in the ER. Remember that *fear* and *pain* are the two things that most frequently interfere with the communication between patient and physician here in the ER. Alleviate or lessen those and your chances of communicating effectively and successfully will be greatly enhanced."

"Today's lecture is about listening." Dr. Rosen turned to the Student and then asked, "Sorry to pick on you, but you're nearby and it's easy for me. One lesson for all of you to learn: Get to lectures early so that you don't have to sit in the front row. It lessens your chances of being called on by the speaker and you won't be noticed as much if you fall asleep. Reminds you of church, doesn't it?" The group again broke into laughter.

"OK, your first trivia question for the day. How fast can the average person speak and how fast can they listen?"

The Student was obviously flustered and despite his best efforts to prevent it, his face turned a fiery red with embarrassment. With some effort he blurted out, "I don't know."

Dr. Rosen smiled and then spoke to the whole group. "Here's your second lesson of the day. Never say 'I don't know.' If they want a number, give them a number. Make something up. Why? Because the person asking for the answer will either think you read it wrong or got confused with some other statistic in your reading. When you answer, 'I don't know,' you remove all doubt of your ignorance." Again, the whole room responded with laughter.

"Now, here's the answer to what you all may be thinking is total trivia—and, believe me, there is a method to my madness. We can speak up to and be understood at about 150 words per minute but we can listen at between 400 and 500 words per minute. Why is it important to know this as we speak to and listen to patients? Anybody?"

A female resident in the back raised her hand timidly, "Is it because our patients can get distracted and their minds wander when we're speaking to them?"

With that, Dr. Rosen reached into the bag, pulled out a miniature Almond Joy candy bar and threw it back to her. "Great answer. That's correct and a perfect lead-in to some of my slides." With that he flipped on the projector and began, "Here's what happens in the communication process. We send a message to someone and we have a certain meaning in mind. The meaning or the content of that message is dependent on our background, emotions, past experience and education to mention just a few things. The other person receives our message but what the person receives is determined by his or her emotional state, background, frame of reference, life experience and education. You can see how easily what is intended to be communicated can be misunderstood by those receiving the message."

"Just think about it. If we can listen about three times faster than the average person speaks, then our minds have all this free time which just lends itself to our tuning out and not hearing the intended message. First question,

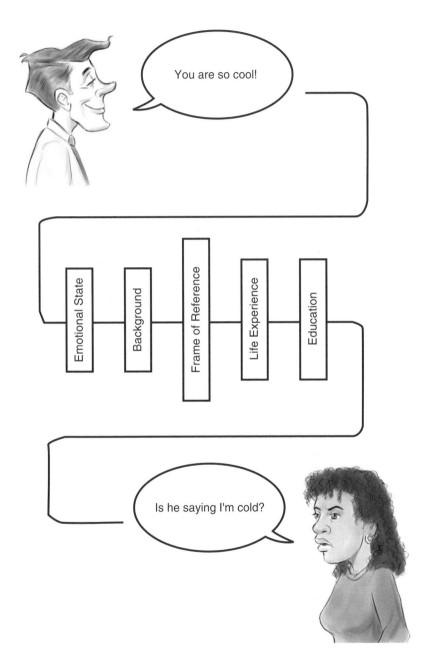

how many potential ways can we send messages when we communicate?"

A male first-year resident said, "Two: one verbally with what we say, and the other with our body language."

An Almond Joy quickly headed his way. "Great! There's one more way in addition to those two ways. It's called paralanguage and it's 'how we say what we say.' Key concept here. **If there's a discrepancy between the verbal and the non-verbal communication, believe the non-verbal.** Let me give you an example. I saw a woman in the ER the other night. She came in complaining of a severe headache. I went in to see her and asked her how she was feeling now as compared to earlier that evening. She answered, 'Fine,' but her body language clearly showed that she was depressed with head down, shoulders sagging and extremely poor affect. If I hadn't looked at the patient when she replied, because I was reading the chart, I would have missed the real meaning behind the actual words that were spoken. It turned out that she had a number of personal issues that were so overwhelming that she developed headaches. We all send many messages when we communicate and part of our job as physicians is to recognize and interpret them correctly.

"We're here today to talk about listening because the most important skill that we possess, as physicians, is the ability to listen to our patients and really hear what they are trying to say to us. You rarely can make a diagnosis if you don't pay attention to what your patients are telling you. Let me take you all back to your first two years of medical school and those exciting basic science lectures that we all were required to attend. Truth be known, I got some of my best sleep in those lectures. First question: How long was your average attention span before your mind started wandering?"

A resident who had been one of Dr. Rosen's advisees in medical school yelled out, "Twenty seconds."

"Loftus, I'm not talking about the total length of time your lovemaking lasts." The class howled at that remark. "Anyone else take a guess?"

One of the medical students guessed next, "Two minutes?"

"Too high, Mahoney, but it might be the length of time you're on this rotation if you don't start wearing socks and a tie. Our patients expect us to look professional even if we don't act that way at times.

"O.K. group, the average length of time that we listen before we start tuning out is about forty seconds. No great surprise since we can listen faster than someone can talk. Next question and I'll do my best Richard Dawson Family Feud imitation for you now, 'Survey says the barriers to effective listening are:'

Barriers to Effective Listening

1. Hop-skip-jump listening. We tune in and out and, as a result, are definitely going to miss important things.
2. Taking too many notes. You'll miss the body language and not hear some of what is said.
3. Dismissing what is being said prematurely and tuning out.
4. Emotionally reacting to sensitive language and not listening. Words with racial overtones, four-letter words or words demeaning to a particular sex may cause us to tune out the speaker because of our reaction to them.
5. Being distracted by the speaker. He or she may be boring, speak in a monotone, use too many technical terms or dress in a distracting manner.
6. Finally, our environment, such as a hard chair, the room being hot, too cold, or too noisy, distracts us.

"My next slide should highlight that last point for you."
The mind can take in only what the ass can endure.
Anyone who had ever been to medical school had to

appreciate that slide and this class was no exception. Every-one clapped heartily in approval.

Dr. Rosen continued with great earnestness. "Think about the environment in the ER or in many patient rooms. They're not private in many cases, they're noisy and the en-vironment is extremely distracting. How well do you think most patients can listen to us—and us to them? Not very. To be successful, it takes work and when you're in pain or afraid or distressed, it's nigh unto impossible to pay atten-tion, as we should. So, it's incumbent upon us all to shape the environment, to keep distractions to a minimum and to repeat what is important to enhance communication.

"Next question. What's the average length of time that goes by before a physician first interrupts a patient after he or she begins speaking? Anyone care to hazard a guess?"

One particularly brave resident raised his hand and replied, "Three minutes?"

Dr. Rosen laughed and said, "If only that were true, our patients would be extremely happy. The average period of time before a physician interrupts a patient is only **eighteen seconds.** It may seem unbelievable to all of you, but keep that number in mind as a reminder before you open your mouth. Questions at this point?"

One of the residents sitting in the back bravely raised her hand. "How can we take the time to listen if the ER is packed and we've got so many patients to see? What you say is all nice in theory but is it really practical to spend some time with each person when patients are stacked everywhere waiting to be seen?"

With her comments, the room got deathly quiet. Dr. Rosen just smiled and said, "Great question that took a lot of guts to ask. I like that in my residents. If we can't back up what we say, then maybe you shouldn't believe us. Keep it up, Dr. Stenger."

The whole room smiled with relief as he continued, "I'm

not saying that you need to take a complete history on every patient. What we all need to do is let the patient tell his or her story before we interrupt. It will only take a minute or so and will immediately help you to direct your questioning and avoid leaping to any premature conclusions. If you screw up because you didn't listen in the beginning, it will take you a lot longer to straighten out any mistakes you might make later. That small investment in time will pay huge dividends later.

"There's a classic study that I believe was put out by the American College of Physicians years ago. As you know, this is not one of those way-out, radical groups, but a group who has a conservative approach to medicine. The study looked at how physicians made a diagnosis. The results were surprising to many, especially younger physicians. The study showed that physicians were able to make a diagnosis almost **70% of the time** simply from the information they got while taking a good clinical history. They used lab tests, X-rays, etc., to help make the diagnosis another 10% to 15% of the time. The hands-on physical exam only helped make the diagnosis about 15% of the time. Remarkable, isn't it? If you needed any proof why we need to listen to patients, then this study surely provides it.

"The next slide is important because of the various cultures that make up our ER patient population. It reads,

Body language and facial expressions are independent of culture.

"Anyone care to tell me what that means?"

One of the residents of Latino heritage raised his hand in response. "Gonzalez, I'll ask you but you'd better know the answer since you're one of my former advisees."

Gonzalez stood up to address the group. "Well, what I think you mean is that regardless of your ethnic background or culture, your body language and facial expressions are universally the same. So, if your face looks angry or surprised, you don't need to know the language because you'll know exactly what the non-verbal clue is telling you. For instance, if for some stupid reason you happened to be walking in my old neighborhood of East L.A., you wouldn't need to know Spanish to know when someone was threatening you or was angry. Anyone could interpret their body language no matter where they're from—even some of my redneck classmates from South Carolina."

Some of the group booed while others just laughed in appreciation.

"Gonzalez, I'm impressed. You're absolutely correct. I couldn't have said it better myself. Here's your Almond Joy.

"O.K. group, I know this is your first rotation and that you might feel a bit overwhelmed at times. Let me assure you that this is the norm and not the exception, despite what some of the more macho types in here might lead the rest of you to believe. Technology can be a pain in the butt at times but there have been some wonderful innovations that have made the physician's life easier.

"I want you to look at my Palm Pilot here. I have it loaded with a few simple programs that have saved me a great deal of time and lessened my likelihood of making mistakes. You can download programs to your Palm that will provide a miniature PDR, a file on potential drug interactions, antibiotic resistance profiles and finally, formulas used to calculate dosages of drugs for children and adults. The beauty of these little PDAs or pocket assistants is it keeps you from having to carry all the reference books around with you. I strongly suggest you explore the benefits of some of these technological innovations for yourself. None of us can remember it all so anything you can do to reduce mistakes can only help you.

"Finally, I'd like to end our session together by telling you a story about a mistake I made early on in my career in the ER that luckily turned out well. I'd gone in to see a forty-one-year-old man who was complaining of chest pain. He worked in construction and looked like he didn't have an ounce of fat on his body. He stated that he occasionally got some pain in his chest and that his wife wanted him to get it checked out. I took a history and the patient had no risk factors except for a father who had an early MI. The patient was unsure of the exact age when it occurred. I did an ECG and it showed no real changes. I figured that it was probably costrochondritis or maybe a muscle strain in the chest that he continued to aggravate. I was about to walk back into the exam room to tell him my very astute diagnosis when one of the older, African-American nurses who had worked in the ER for longer than my actual age at the time stopped me with a question.

"Dr. Rosen, have you talked to the family members about your patient yet?" My very learned response was, "No, hadn't planned on it as the problem seems pretty straightforward to me.

"The nurse just stared at me for a minute, shook her head, gave a little frown and said, 'You know old Mary here ain't gonna be around here forever to be training you young doctors and helping to pull your bacon out of the fire at times. Honey, if you don't mind listening to an old lady, make sure you always talk to the family before you ever make your final diagnosis. You'll learn one hell of a lot about the real problem that your patient might have and not just what's written on the ER chart when they come in. Now your young man in there has got a pretty little wife out in the waiting room who's as nervous as a cat on a hot tin roof, and keeps asking to talk to her husband's doctor. If I were you, honey, I'd go talk to her right now.'

"Fortunately for me, my ego that day didn't get in the way of my listening to Mrs. Mary Brown, that seventy-two-year-old nurse. Instead of going into the patient's room, I went instead to the waiting room to speak to his wife and then, as Paul Harvey used to say, I got 'the rest of the story.'

"What I learned from his wife was that this very healthy appearing young man had such severe chest pain at times that he would stop whatever he was doing and clutch his chest with a clenched fist in the classical sign of someone with angina. I also discovered that he not only had a father who had an MI at an early age but had one uncle who died in his forties of a heart attack and had two brothers who had bypass surgery in their early forties. I called the medical man on call and got the patient admitted to the CCU. He had a stress test the next morning that was so positive that he had an emergency cath that afternoon. The catheterization showed a 95% blockage of the LAD and at least an 80% block of the right artery and the circumflex. For you students here, the LAD or left anterior descending coronary artery is referred to as the 'Widowmaker.' Anyone have any idea why?"

One of the female medical students eagerly raised her hand. "They call it the 'Widowmaker' because it supplies more blood to the muscle of the heart than any other coronary artery. If that gets blocked off completely, then it's likely that the heart will suffer so much damage that the person will die."

"Excellent answer. Unfortunately, many people have no warning signs, such as the chest pain of angina to tell them that they're not getting enough blood flow to the heart, so they end up having that fatal heart attack, when having a stress test would likely have detected the problem. To finish my story, the patient of mine had triple-vessel bypass surgery two days after I saw him in the ER. As you all can understand now, I would have missed a potentially fatal diagnosis if I first hadn't listened to my nurse. My take-home lesson for you all is to involve family members in all your ultimate treatment plans.

"In that same vein, now might be a good time for me to review some of the simple rules that I'll be preaching to all of you over the next few years. Use them and you increase your chances of a successful patient encounter.

1. Introduce yourself with a SMILE and then address the person as Mr., Mrs. or Miss and not by his or her first names.
2. Always explain to patients what's going to happen to them.
3. Drape the person so that there is a minimum of bodily exposure and always have a chaperone if working with a member of the opposite sex.
4. Always thank the patient when you are done.
5. Always include the family in your discussions but only after you get the patient's permission.
6. Before leaving, answer any questions and write down any instructions for follow-up care, such as how to take medicines or who should be seen in follow-up and when.

"These seem like simple things but they are overlooked more times than not by students, residents and experienced physicians, even the faculty at our esteemed medical institution. It's simple courtesy . . . nothing more than that."

Dr. Rosen clapped his hands, gave them all a big smile and said, "Thanks for listening this morning. Now it's time to go stamp out disease and save some lives. Remember, we've been given a gift to be doing what we do, so enjoy yourselves. Come see me if I can help you in any way. Now get out of here."

The Student left and went to the ER where he was assigned to spend the next week with a third-year resident and the Pediatric attending, Dr. Nancy Cummings. He was surprised, and a bit upset, to learn that the resident he'd been assigned to, Dr. Humphrey, was also a female.

"Just my luck, two women. I hope they don't start talking about all this touchy-feely crap. I just want to learn how to do some pro-

cedures and try to avoid as many screaming brats as I can. Why the pediatrics side of the ER, right out of the box? God, that would be my hell on earth if I had to take care of kids full-time."

The first patient they went to see was a nine-year-old boy who complained of an ankle injury after falling off his skateboard while trying to do some tricks. The resident examined the ankle; all the while explaining to the Student what she was doing and what she discovered. She then asked the Student to do the same. When they were done, she explained to the little boy that they'd be getting an X-ray and when that was done, they'd be back.

Because the ER was one of the busiest in the city, it took almost forty-five minutes before the patient was back with his X-ray in hand. The resident reviewed the film in front of the patient and his mother and again explained to the Student what he should look for when looking at an ankle film. Fortunately, the ankle was not broken but merely sprained, which meant that some of the ligaments had been stretched and partially torn. The resident then put the Student on the spot with a question, "O.K., what are you going to tell our patient to do so that he gets back on his skateboard as soon as possible?"

The Student could feel himself getting red in the face with embarrassment. The resident's question had caught him completely off guard. He was enjoying just listening to her and hadn't expected to be put on the spot yet. "Well, when I hurt my ankle playing basketball a few times, I put ice on it and wrapped it for a few days. That seemed to get the swelling down quite a bit."

"Great, that's part of what we'll do. One easy thing for all patients to remember is what we call RICE. It stands for Rest, Ice, Compression and Elevation. Our little friend here needs to get off his ankle so that he doesn't injure it more, so we'll give him some crutches for a few days. That's the rest part of RICE.

"Next, he'll need to put an ice pack on the injured part of the ankle for at least fifteen minutes every few hours for the first couple of days. The ice helps to stop the bleeding inside that occurs when the ligaments get torn. When the ice is applied, it should be done with an Ace wrap, putting some pressure on the area. When the ice pack is taken off, the ankle should be wrapped—or compressed—so the swelling is less and so that the ankle doesn't move. Any movement will cause more bleeding inside the ankle and more stretching of the injured ligaments.

"Finally, since we are resting the ankle for a few days, we'll also elevate it on a pillow or two while he's sitting or in bed. Do you know why we do this?"

Again, the Student had no clue. "No, I'm not sure."

"Elevating the ankle, or any swollen or injured joint for that matter, helps the blood to drain out of the area. When you injure the ankle, you damage the veins and lymphatic vessels that help return blood to the heart. These take a few weeks to heal and it's one of the reasons the ankle remains swollen for weeks or months after an injury. If you don't tell patients, or their parents in this case, about what to expect, they'll often get worried and think something may be wrong when, in fact, it's a normal part of the healing process.

"Let me give you a personal experience. When I was in college, I hurt my ankle while playing soccer one day. It wasn't broken but the ER doctor I saw that night told me little or nothing about what to expect. I panicked the next day when I saw blood all around my ankle that only worsened the following day. He hadn't told me that this was normal as the blood from the injured veins and arteries around the ligament pooled around the ankle area. I ran back to my team physician who explained that this was normal and that the body takes time to heal itself, but that it would all go away in time."

Without anyone noticing, Dr. Cummings had slipped into the room and spoke at that point, "One thing you'll hear over and over in medicine is the phrase 'The Tincture of Time.' It simply means that given enough time, the body will often heal itself, provided that the physician doesn't do anything rash or stupid to interfere. Nice job explaining things, Dr. Humphrey."

"Thanks. Now I'm going to show Mom and our patient how to properly wrap an ankle. I learned this from Dr. Cummings when I was a resident. I thought I knew how to do something as simple as wrapping an ankle but I was doing it all wrong and it really makes a huge difference when you do it right. Now when you wrap the ankle or any extremity, always wrap from the outermost, or distal, portion to the inner portion so that the swelling is forced toward the heart. Make sure there are no wrinkles in the Ace wrap so the skin doesn't get damaged, and do it in figure-eight fashion for more support and strength." The resident then smiled at the little boy. "Since you'll be elevating this, it will help to reduce the swelling considerably. Loosen it for ten minutes a few times a day and then rewrap it. After a few days, you can begin walking on the ankle again. Then I like to switch to this Aircast. It fits right inside your tennis shoe and is hardly noticeable. An Aircast is often used by athletes to prevent further injury and to help them return to normal activity sooner. Like I said, you'll notice some swelling for several weeks but that will go away in time. Oh, almost forgot, you'll notice some red and blue blood under the skin around the ankle in a day or so and it can last for weeks. Nothing to be alarmed about—but if I didn't warn you about it, you might panic and think I'd missed something. O.K., any questions?"

She's good, the Student thought. *I didn't know any of this stuff and I sure thought I knew how to take care of an ankle sprain and how to wrap an ankle. Maybe I can learn a few things that might be useful here.*

Dr. Cummings stuck her head back into the room and

asked of the resident, "Can I borrow your Student for a few minutes? I've got something I want him to see."

"Sure, we're just about finished here anyway."

Dr. Cummings led the Student to another exam room down the hall. At the door she stopped and explained, "There's a little twelve-month-old girl in here who's been sick for a few days with a fever, URI symptoms and lethargy. The mother thinks she's getting worse despite the use of OTC medicines including anti-pyretics. I've examined the little girl and done some basic lab work. I can't find a ready source for the infection she's obviously got so I'm going to have to do a spinal tap on her. I thought you might want to see it."

"Thanks, I would. I've never seen one done before."

They entered the room together and Dr. Cummings introduced the Student to the mother who had obviously been crying. "I have a little girl of my own at home and so I understand how the idea of the spinal tap can be so upsetting. Let me assure you that your child will not be in pain. She'll likely begin crying because we are going to have to restrain her so she can't get loose, and not because we're doing anything to hurt her. You're welcome to stay but I think you'll do better if you don't have to watch. I'll come get you when I'm done. O.K.?"

The mother nodded her head to indicate yes in a very resigned fashion. She didn't like what was going to happen to her baby but knew it was for the best. She slowly left the room but only after talking to her little girl and giving her a goodbye kiss.

The nurse working with Dr. Cummings quickly wrapped the little girl in a sheet and turned her on her side with her bare back facing Dr. Cummings' stool. The doctor sat on the stool and then put on her sterile gloves. She unwrapped the LP, or lumbar puncture tray, and arranged the instruments. She then began her explanation. "We're going to swab the back with some Betadine to disinfect the skin. This way when we put the LP needle through the skin, it will lessen the chances of introducing bacteria into the spinal fluid. We don't want to cause problems with this procedure. We let this dry for a minute and then we're ready to numb the skin over where we insert the needle as well as the area underneath the skin." Dr. Cummings showed the Student how to draw up the local anesthetic and how to make a little wheal on the skin before going deeper. She then showed him how to put together the LP needle and the manometer for measuring the spinal fluid pressure once they were in the spinal canal.

"O.K., folks, here we go. We slide the needle slowly between the vertebrae and we aim for the umbilicus. It makes it easier to do this when your assistant bends the patient's back like our wonderful nurse, Millie, is doing. As you go in you will feel the needle meet some slight resistance and then you'll feel a pop as it enters the spinal canal. There we go. We should be in now." Dr. Cummings pulled out the safety hub of the needle and almost immediately a drop of clear liquid appeared at the end of the needle. Before it could fall out, she hooked the manometer to the needle and measured the pressure, which was normal. Then, she began to collect the spinal fluid in three separate tubes so that it could be sent to the lab for various tests.

"This looks very good on initial appearances. It's clear like water and that's a good sign. Kids with meningitis often have cloudy spinal fluid that is under some increased pressure. This is slow coming out which is another good sign. Let's hope my initial impressions are correct. Now, I want you to slowly pull out the needle for me so you can feel it come out through the various tissue levels. Once it's out, I want you to rub the spot in a circular fashion to help prevent any further spinal fluid from leaking out. Finally, put on a Band-Aid and we'll be done."

When they were finished, they picked up the little girl and took her with them to assure her mother that everything had turned out fine. After they had spoken to the mother for a few minutes and were returning to the front desk, the overhead speaker blared out the message that got everyone's heartbeat racing. "Code Blue, emergency room. Code Blue, emergency room." It was the hospital's internal code for a cardiac arrest and meant that the cardiopulmonary resuscitation, or CPR team, should respond to the location named—ASAP. The noise level in the ER had picked up immediately and the sound of running feet seemed to be all around them.

Dr. Cummings immediately quickened her pace. "Let's go, Student. Stick with me on this one. Stay in the corner out of the way and watch the action. We'll talk about it later."

They got to the ER's main desk and were immediately directed to the trauma room, "EMS just brought in a man in an MVA who arrested as they pulled up to the back door."

One of the attendings on the trauma side of the ER was already present and beginning to bark out orders to the assembled group. The most senior person at an arrest usually directed the resuscitation efforts unless a person's personal physician was present. The key to any successful CPR effort was restoring blood flow and oxygenation as soon as possible, because in only seven minutes without blood flow to the brain, permanent damage would occur. Seconds could mean the difference between success and failure.

There was blood all over the patient and his blood pressure was extremely low. In a trauma patient, this usually meant that he had lost a great deal of blood and if doctors could get enough fluids into the patient to increase his BP, then they might be able to get the heart going long enough to find the source of bleeding, and then get the patient to emergency surgery to stop it.

The Student was clearly stunned and couldn't take it all in. Doctors and nurses were intubating the patient, starting IV fluids in multiple sites, pounding up and down on the patient's chest, removing his clothes and inserting a catheter into his bladder—all at the same time. He had never seen so much activity and so much yelling at one time.

Holy Christ! This whole scene reminds me of a scene from an African safari travelogue in which a herd of hyenas had attacked a zebra. They had darted in and out, each taking their turn at the defenseless zebra, much like the patient on the table was with the pack of ER attendants. It was almost surreal.

As the IV fluids were pumped into the patient, the blood pressure slowly began to rise and the normal heart rhythm was restored. The energy level in the room fell dramatically but the Student's heartbeat continued to race as he watched the scene unfold in front of him. He almost jumped through the ceiling when Dr. Cummings touched his arm to indicate it was time to leave the room. When they got into the hall, a couple of ER residents were already talking about the patient.

"What do you think the chances are of our man making it?"

"Pretty damn good now. In young people with good hearts, they have a good chance of surviving once they stop the bleeding. Now his biggest risk is kidney shutdown, internal bleeding or infection from all his trauma."

Dr. Cummings jumped in at that point. "What do you think your chances are of making it, Dr. Park?"

"Uh, I don't know what you mean?"

"What I mean is that you both are idiots. You're in there doing CPR on a man with blood and body fluids everywhere and you're not even close to following universal barrier protection guidelines. You ever hear of HIV or hepatitis, not to mention a number of other diseases easily communicated from our patients? Do you remember that article I mentioned by Caplan in which one of four of their trauma patients had a transmissible disease? Frankly, I'm really pissed. Neither of you wore masks or gowns during the resuscitation. Many of the others did the same and some of the nurses didn't even wear protective glasses. Don't get me wrong. We're not unique. In a recent study in the *Southern Medical Journal*, the percentage of healthcare workers wearing barrier protection other than gloves was considerably less than 50%. And don't give me that 'I didn't have time' bullcrap, as it just doesn't float my boat. Next time, I will embarrass you in front of the whole team. Do I make myself clear?"

The two residents sheepishly nodded their heads in assent. Dr. Cummings then turned to go back to the Pediatric side of the house with the Student. As they walked, she said, "It only takes one slip-up or one needle stick to transmit a potentially fatal or life-altering disease. There's always time to put on a gown or a pair of glasses. Oh, that reminds me, have you gotten your Hep A and Hep B immunizations?"

The Student knew she was angry and didn't want any of that flowing downhill to him so he was glad to be able to say, "Yes, I finished the series this past month."

"Great, now let's go see some patients."

Thankfully, the remainder of the day was uneventful so the Student left the ER after his eight-hour shift and headed for the third-year study carrels in the basement of the hospital. He couldn't believe how drained and tired he felt. He'd survived his first day. At the same time he felt exhilarated because he'd learned more than he ever thought possible in one day. Most importantly, he had gained a great deal of practical knowledge that he could use to really treat patients. It was so different from the basic science years. He felt like his real medical education was now underway. He soon met some of his classmates who were also finishing their days on their first rotations. He spotted one of his friends with whom he often played pickup basketball, and immediately began to tell him about his day and what he'd learned. Soon the stories of the day were flying everywhere. This sharing among peers was one of the oldest forms of both teaching and learning and would continue for the rest of the Student's medical career in some fashion or another.

✤ *Perspectives for Doctors* ✤

Medical interviewing is an enormously complex task. Doctor-patient communication has a direct impact on patient satisfaction, compliance with treatment and ultimately, on the final clinical outcome. Physicians must in a **fifteen-minute visit** determine symptoms, make diagnoses, get to know the patient's psychosocial situation, develop a therapeutic relationship and counsel the patient about behaviors and therapies. Are you kidding me? With expectations like those, are we doomed to failure? Definitely not, but to be successful, it takes a special effort and a genuine caring attitude.

Truly listening to anyone is hard work. As mentioned previously, you can listen faster than the other person can talk so it's extremely easy to get distracted by your own thoughts, by the surroundings, or by the message and mannerisms of the sender to mention a few listening distractions. Think back to when you were in school and how much easier it was for you to daydream than to listen to the particular point the teacher was trying to make. No matter how good a speaker someone is, it's extremely hard to hold someone else's attention for more than a few minutes at a time.

Now think about the situation in which a physician might find herself. She's got a crowded office. She's behind and just had a fight with one of the managed care organizations about a patient. Her spouse is upset because one of the kids is sick with a temperature and one of their aging parents is not doing well physically. Do you think she's got a few distractions in the way of really listening to patients? You bet she does. Physicians are only human.

Patients may have some of the same issues affecting their ability to hear what physicians are trying to say as well. They may not like the message or the diagnosis that we've just given. They might be distracted by pain or other medical problems they are having. They might be so upset by the manner of the physician or his staff that they are not hearing what is really being said. So many things can interfere with the communication process. The trick to improving all this is fairly simple but also requires staying in the moment. The secret to listening success is called **Active Listening.**

Here's how active listening works. If you are listening to someone speak to you, you must repeat back what he said to you before you can answer him. If you don't get his message correct, then he must repeat it again and you must then repeat it—until you get it correctly. He must then do the same with what you told him before he can speak. It becomes somewhat tedious at first but, before long, people are really listening intently to what you are trying to say. Here's an example of how this listening technique works.

You and your wife are talking and you agree to use active listening to improve your communication. She is trying to tell you that she had a really bad day at the office and that she had a run-in with her boss.

You reply, "What I heard you saying was that you had a bad day at work and that you'd really like to quit your job. Is that correct?"

She says, "No, it's not. I said that I had a bad day but I never said anything about quitting. That was your way of trying to solve today's bad day for me."

You reply, "So you had a bad day. Sounds like it got you really mad. What are you feeling inside?"

She says, "My day was bad. Thanks for listening and caring about how I feel. I'm feeling very mad at the moment because my boss doesn't appreciate all that I do at the office. I think that he takes me for granted a lot of the time."

You say, "You're feeling pretty frustrated about not being

appreciated. Is that right?" (Head nods yes.) "Is there anything that I can do to help?"

She says, "You are concerned and want to help. No, I don't need for you to do anything. I just wanted you to listen. It makes me feel so special when you do. Thanks. I love you, dear." (You now get a great big "attaboy" from your wife who feels really understood. Congratulations! You've just learned the value of Active Listening).

Now how does this work with any part of your life?

1. **If you want someone to listen better, then make sure that he repeats back what you intended before he can ask a question or interrupt.**
2. **If the other person won't change his habits and do better, then be prepared to walk away until he does. The real power that you have is your ability to opt out of a relationship until the other person is willing to work at it and listen.**

In the doctor-patient relationship, either party has the ability to discharge the other. Physicians do not have to deal with disruptive, non-compliant patients and patients do not have to deal with physicians who will not listen to their concerns. If enough people take this action, then it can make a difference.

Practice active listening in all areas of your life. It will not only help communication with those you care about, but will certainly ensure a better understanding of what patients are trying to communicate. It's not easy but it's well worth the extra effort. May I suggest that we all keep the old Chinese proverb in mind, "*Because God has given us two ears and one mouth, we should listen twice as much as we speak.*

The Doctor as Detective

The Advisor turned slowly in his chair and looked at the Student for a moment before speaking. "Have you ever heard of Sherlock Holmes, Fr. Brown or Hercule Poirot, Student?"

"Of course, I've heard of Sherlock Holmes but I've got no clue about those other guys."

"Very punny, Student, even if you didn't realize it! Fr. Brown was the principal character in mystery stories written by G.K. Chesterton. Hercule Poirot was the featured detective in a number of books authored by Agatha Christie. You have at least heard of Agatha Christie, haven't you?"

"Sure, I have. I just didn't know who Hercules Pwat Rot was."

The Advisor slowly shook his head in disbelief while muttering, "God help us, but where have the liberal arts gone! I guess this is going to take a bit longer than I expected. Do you have any idea why I asked you about all these famous detectives, especially Sherlock Holmes?"

It's a real mystery to me, laughed the Student to himself. *Is this a trick question? What could this possibly have to do with learning about medicine? The old guy is really out there now,* he thought. *It looks like it's going to be a long afternoon again.*

"I can see from the puzzled look on your face that the light's on but no one's at home," chuckled the Advisor.

Somewhat wearily he went on. "Sherlock Holmes was one of the most famous detectives in literature and was created by Sir Arthur Conan Doyle, who himself was a physician.

The character Sherlock Holmes was a wonderful observer of life in general, and of people in particular. In solving the various crimes presented to him, he always made some astute observation about people or the facts that everyone else had missed. They were, in fact, very simple observations, but by putting them all together into a total picture, he was able to make sense of things and solve a seemingly unsolvable mystery. The fun and fascinating part for everyone who reads the stories is trying to figure out all this before Conan Doyle reveals it to you in the story."

The Advisor got up and began to pace back and forth slowly, talking all the while.

"It's believed that Sir Arthur . . . you know he was knighted by the Queen for his achievements . . . based the Sherlock Holmes character on another English physician, Dr. John Bell. Today's reading assignment is a short essay written by Dr. Bell that highlights beautifully the need for close observation of people and life as part of being a good doctor. When you've finished this, call me and we'll meet in the surgery clinic. And Student, wear your white coat."

Within the hour, the Student was down in the surgery clinic. As always, the clinic was a zoo. There were many patients moving through it each day, either being evaluated for surgery or in follow-up after surgery. Today's clinic was orthopedic surgery, and it was no exception. There were people everywhere. Everyone seemed to be either on crutches, or wearing a brace or sling on one of their appendages.

The Advisor and Student met by the front desk and before they did anything the Advisor asked, "What are the two happiest years of an orthopedist's life, Student?"

"Uh . . . internship and chief residency?"

"No, it's second grade," laughed the Advisor. "The joke is

Sherlock Holmes, the doctor.

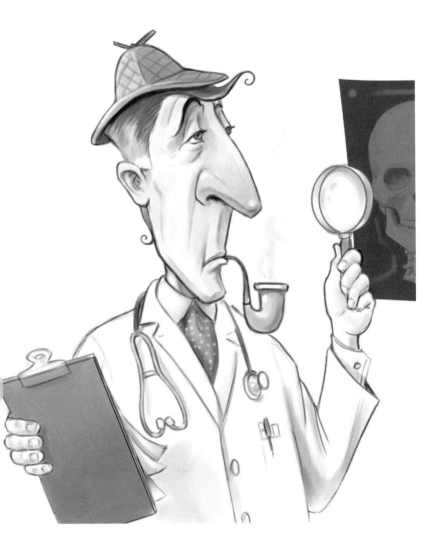

that orthopods have the reputation of not being the brightest bulbs on the porch. My brother is an orthopedist in Charlotte, North Carolina, and I so like to tease him with jokes about his specialty. He's a brilliant, compassionate doctor but the image of orthopedists in general is not helped by the type of surgery they do. It's been compared to being a carpenter because a lot of it can often be fairly mechanical with lots of saws, lathes and heavy grunt work. This, coupled with all the ex-jocks who've gone into orthopedics, doesn't improve their perception by others. I personally don't think their reputation is deserved, but you'll have to make that decision for yourself.

"O.K., what we're going to do today is to begin working on your own powers of observation. You and I are going to see a patient together. Then I'll ask you some questions about what you've seen. Sound fair?"

"I guess so," the Student said cautiously.

The Advisor beckoned to another doctor wearing surgical scrubs covered by a dirty white lab coat. "Hey, Paul, this is my advisee I told you about. Have you got a couple of patients for us to see?"

"I sure do and they've all agreed to speak to you both. I've got the charts over here on this desk. Our group has already seen each of them so they're free to go when you're finished. They were more than happy to wait for a few minutes and play a part in your student's education."

"Thanks, Paul, I really appreciate your help," the Advisor said as he scooped up the patient charts.

The Advisor and Student entered the nearest room and introduced themselves to a middle-aged man wearing a golf shirt, tan pants, and a pair of slip-on shoes. The Advisor succinctly explained their purpose and then asked, "How long have you been bothered by arthritis?"

"Three years, but thanks to Celebrex, things are a lot more

tolerable lately," the patient said as he rubbed his knee unconsciously.

"Mr. Goryance, I'd like to ask my Student a few questions about you so that he can test his powers of observation. Then I'll tell him what I think I've observed. Finally, we'll ask you to tell us both what the correct answer is. Would that be O.K. with you?"

"Sure, no problem. Sounds interesting."

"Great! Here's the first question. What does Mr. Goryance like to do for fun?"

The Student stared back at the Advisor with a blank stare.

Where is he coming from? I've never seen this guy before and haven't gotten to ask him even a single question, so how am I supposed to know what he does for fun? Who knows, maybe he writes mystery stories like some of those other guys he told me about?

"Work in his garden?" the Student guessed.

"I don't think so . . . but he might. I'm going to guess that he likes to play golf for fun. Is that right, Mr. Goryance?"

"Right you are, Doc, but how'd you know? It's not in my chart."

"Elementary my dear Watson . . . or Goryance, in this case. A few things gave it away. You have a tan that ends slightly above your ankles so I assumed that you must wear those little footsie socks that many golfers use during the summer. Your left hand is much less tan than your right. This is usually found in right-handed golfers because they wear their golf gloves on their non-dominant hands. The final clue was your golf shirt with the name Pebble Beach embroidered on it. Only serious golfers will usually pay the huge greens fees it takes to play on that course. You put all these things together and it didn't take much guesswork to know you were a regular golfer."

"Pretty impressive, Doc," said Mr. Goryance with some awe.

"Thanks," the Advisor said with a smile, "and now it's on to the second question. Looking at Mr. Goryance, I can tell that he's obviously had cancer, Student. Can you tell me what type, and what he can do to prevent it in the future?"

The Student's mind raced but despite his best efforts he couldn't come up with even a guess at what kind of cancer Mr. Goryance could have had. He was still amazed at the first bit of detective work. It seemed so simple when the Advisor had explained how he came to his conclusion after the fact, but he felt stupid for missing every one of those clues.

"I can see by the look on your face that you'd only be guessing, so let me tell you what I believe I've observed. One of the hazards that Mr. Goryance faces as a golfer is sun exposure. This puts him at increased risk for skin cancer especially on the area of his body where most people forget to use sun block: the ears. I can see by looking at the small scars on his face, neck and arms that he's had numerous skin cancers removed. He's obviously fair skinned so this puts him at an even higher risk for skin cancer than darker skinned individuals."

The Advisor turned to Mr. Goryance to confirm what he said was true. An amazed look was on his face and he could only nod his head in agreement. "What should Mr. Goryance do now to prevent, or lessen, his chances of skin cancer in the future?"

The Student paused for only a few seconds before replying. "He should use a sun block with an SPF of at least 30 whenever he goes outside . . . even on cloudy days, since you can still be exposed to ultraviolet rays on those days. He should consider using a hat when outdoors, and he should have annual skin exams by his physician to detect potential trouble spots before they turn into actual cancers. I believe these are called AK's or actinic keratoses. Finally, and one of the most important things he should do, would be to examine his own skin at home regularly to detect the early signs of the same recurrent skin cancers he's been having. He should also look for the early warning signs of the most dangerous type of skin cancer, malignant melanoma, because he's at increased risk of this due to his past history of sun exposure."

The Student paused and looked anxiously at his Advisor.

"Fantastic, I couldn't have said that any better. You've obviously learned that lesson well. That's exactly what you need to teach to all your patients who work or play out in the sun. It's even more important to tell children and young people as they tend to overdo the exposure more and aren't as careful about using sun block. Many experts believe it's a bad sunburn early in life that puts you at risk for skin cancer later in life. Mr. Goryance, do you take all those precautions now?"

"No, I sure don't, but you can bet I will in the future. I had no idea the sun could cause all the damage your student mentioned. Is it really important?"

"Mr. Goryance, it may just save your life one day. Melanoma is a deadly cancer but the cure rate is over 95% if caught early enough—so yes, what my student told you is extremely important, and I would follow his advice if I were you."

With that the Advisor smiled, extended his hand to Mr. Goryance and said, "Thanks so much for giving us your time and helping us learn. I'm trying to help my Student discover how, by developing his powers of observation, he will learn so much more about each patient and better care for the total patient."

They left that room and immediately moved to the next where a middle-aged, thin, African-American woman was sitting on the exam table. She had a half smile on her face and was leaning forward, breathing in and out through somewhat pursed lips. The Advisor made the introductions and again explained the reason for their being there.

"I want you to take a look at Mrs. Rhinehardt for a minute. Then I want you to move closer and examine her eyes. After you're done, I want you to tell me four important, potentially life-affecting diagnoses you can make about her by just looking closely."

Life-affecting diagnoses? All I see is some old woman who reminds me a little bit of the actress Cicely Tyson. Gosh, she was good in that old movie about civil rights. Christ, that reminds me that I'm supposed to take Christine to see "Erin Brockovich" at the movies tonight and I haven't even told her what time. Jeez, I'd better get back to reality and start concentrating on Mrs. R. or my ass is grass and my Advisor is a lawnmower.

The Student moved closer to the patient and looked carefully at her eyes. He did note numerous areas of tanned, raised, soft appearing, globular growths on either side of the lateral aspect of her eyes. He remembered reading about them in one of his clinical texts. "The patient looks like she . . ."

"Stop right there, Student. The patient has a name and it's Mrs. Rhinehardt. We, as physicians, have the privilege of caring for patients and learning from them. They deserve our respect. As such, we should always use a person's name when we are talking about him or her. Got it?"

The Student, looking somewhat ashamed, nodded affirmatively.

"O.K., now go on."

"Well, uh, Mrs. Rhinehardt has some skin lesions close to her eyes that can be associated with high cholesterol. I also noted that she has some similar areas near her elbows. Therefore, I'm going to guess that one of her life altering diagnoses is high cholesterol. If she does have high cholesterol, then she's at increased risk of heart disease." The Student stopped and looked again at the patient before continuing, "I hate to admit it but I really can't find the other three things you must have noticed."

"Good pickup on the skin lesions. They are associated

with the increased cholesterol you mentioned, and you're right, they can be a clue to an increased risk of heart disease. Now, the other things that I observed in Mrs. Rhinehardt are severely deformed finger joints on both hands that are consistent with rheumatoid arthritis. I also noticed some yellowing of the index and middle fingers on her right hand which likely means that she's a heavy smoker. It's harder to see in African-Americans but Mrs. Rhinehardt is extremely fair-skinned, so it's a bit easier to detect on her. The final thing that I noticed is the one medical problem having the greatest negative impact on her life . . . and it's closely related to her heavy smoking. She has chronic obstructive pulmonary disease, or COPD. You can tell this by the way she breathes. She has the characteristic appearance of what was once called a 'pink puffer.' She leans forward when breathing while at the same time pursing her lips. Persons with COPD do this to lessen the resistance in their airways so that they move air in and out of their lungs easier. Did we miss anything, Mrs. Rhinehardt?"

"No, doctor, you and the other doctor got all my medical problems right. You were also right when you talked about my breathing problem. It is the thing that distresses me the most. It keeps me from doing the things that I want to do in life . . . even the simplest of things. I have to stop to catch my breath just walking up the few stairs to my house. I can't do housework like I used to, and I can't even play with my grandkids. I got two of them and I can't hardly do anything with them. I should have stopped smoking years ago but I'm so addicted to those damn cigarettes," she said with an embarrassed smile.

The Advisor thanked Mrs. Rhinehardt for her honesty and openness and then helped her off the examining table. They all left the room together. As they watched the woman move slowly down the hall, the Advisor turned and spoke with obvious sadness in his voice. "Having COPD and/or emphysema is a horrible way to live, but an even more horrible way to die. She's a brave person but, as she aptly said, those damn cigarettes have taken their toll.

"Student, I know you must be feeling discouraged about all you missed. Believe me, you didn't do badly for your first time at this. I felt the same way after my first encounter with my advisor, Dr. Clifton Meador. He taught me so much about the Art of Medicine and about caring for patients. You'll get better and better at it but only if you keep trying and take the time to really look at your patients. It's like any other skill. It can be learned, but only if you're willing to take time and work at it. It's so easy to become focused in on one system, one part of the body, or one diagnosis, and miss lots of other clues that help provide insights into your patient. The more you can observe and know about your patient, the better the care you can provide. Remember the article I had you read last week by Dr. Newburg? He asked one of the most important questions that we all face when we set a goal for ourselves. Are you really willing to work hard enough to attain it? Many people say they are, but just don't follow through. 'The spirit is often willing but the flesh is weak' that quote from the Bible pretty well characterizes the human condition in so many ways."

The Advisor paused and just shook his head. "Enough philosophizing for today. Think about what you've learned. I know you can do it. I have faith in you, and after all, you have me to help you." The Advisor laughed heartily at his comment, clapped the Student on the back and headed back to his office.

I am discouraged, the Student thought. *How can I ever pick up on things the way my Advisor did? Was he really as bad as I was today when he first started? It's hard for me to believe that. I saw a few piddly things but missed so many obvious clues.*

He reflected back on the two encounters and was again impressed by the way his Advisor had noticed so many things about the patients and how he did so in only a few minutes. He hadn't even asked a single question. The Student knew he had a lot to learn but seeing these two patients with his Advisor gave him some new insights into how to approach other patients. He vowed to begin looking at every patient encounter like a detective . . . like the famous Sherlock Holmes. Heck, he might even begin reading some of those mystery stories the Advisor talked about.

Maybe I can change? He wondered.

✣ *Perspectives for Doctors* ✣

They've been called "disease detectives," "medical sleuths," and the "medical CIA." Their real name is the Epidemic Intelligence Service or EIS. To quote an article in the April 2001, issue of the *Journal of the American Medical Association* (*JAMA*), "They're perhaps the most influential medical group you've never heard of" and they're celebrating fifty years of existence. They've investigated and solved some of the most serious and life-threatening infectious disease problems all over the world. Their investigations include the first case of AIDS, polio and smallpox outbreaks, Legionnaire's disease, Ebola virus, toxic shock syndrome and West Nile virus. The EIS program was originally designed to detect and stop epidemics of disease but now deals primarily with prevention of various occupational, environmental and worldwide health problems. Sherlock Holmes is alive and well and now can be found working on medical cases in all parts of the world.

Contrary to what most people would like to believe, medicine is often not black and white, but many shades of gray. Most patients don't present with the classic symptoms of a particular disease. Instead, they may have only one or two symptoms of a problem and it's the physician's job to figure out the real problem. It's only when the patient shares all his or her signs and symptoms with the physician that the physician can decipher what the correct diagnosis might be from a variety of possibilities. For example, a patient might come to the doctor complaining of fatigue and weakness. There's a long list of possible diagnoses that have these general complaints and included are hepatitis, diabetes, viral illnesses, AIDS, thyroid disorders, cancer and a host of other problems. It's only when the physician applies her interviewing skills to the patient's problem that she can begin to deduce the problem. One of the most revealing statistics that I've seen (and is unknown to many) is that a diagnosis can be made almost **70%** of the time by a skilled physician, just by talking to a patient and taking a history. This is a mind-boggling figure. All it requires is taking time with the patient to listen and ask the right questions. Because the doctor-patient relationship is a two way street, it also takes a patient who is honest and shares openly with his physician for the entire story to come out. This requires time and trust. Some of the more uncommon diagnoses take time to decipher so patients must learn to be patient as well. Many medical conditions do **not** present with symptoms specific to that disease but rather present with signs and symptoms generic to many problems.

Making the correct diagnosis is like being a detective. You look at the clues and are led down certain paths based on those clues. Sometimes, it's the correct path and sometimes it's not. Many diseases may present similarly initially, and only over a period of time does the particular disease a patient may have present characteristics that allow its proper diagnosis. Two very important longstanding adages in medicine are applicable in working up a particular medical problem. The first is, **"When you hear hoof-beats, you don't think of zebras,"** which is closely related to **"In medicine, common things occur most commonly."**

If you hear hoof-beats, you think of horses because it's the

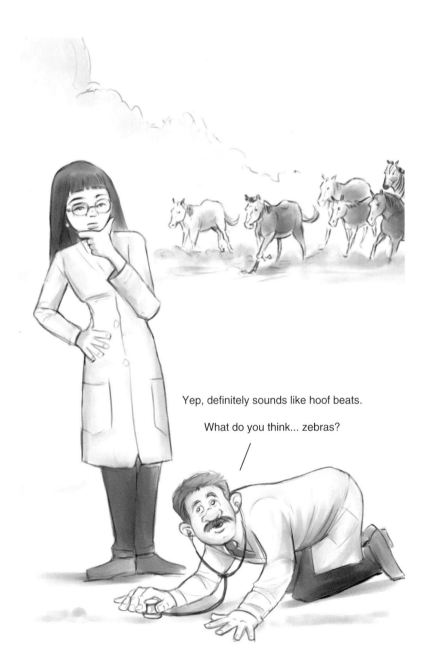

most common thing. When a patient presents with fever, shaking chills and a headache, you think of the flu or a cold and you don't think of some rare tropical disease. We treat a person for the common problem or illness and we'll be correct ninety-nine times out of a hundred. You don't routinely think to ask a patient of travel to an exotic area when you see him or her for an illness with cold-like symptoms, especially during the wintertime. However, a patient could have just returned from Africa and could have malaria, but the chances are extremely rare. The physician may miss this because it's not a common problem, one that we routinely encounter. Physicians are generally so pressed for time that they don't waste time asking extraneous questions, so it is important to give them any pertinent changes in a patient's situation. We have to assume the norm.

This brings me to the next medical adage: **"Give every problem the Tincture of Time."** Almost every illness has a period of time before a patient's immune system kicks in and you start seeing improvement. Give illnesses time to run their course before jumping in and doing something stupid that can make things worse. The body is a miraculous instrument designed to heal itself (in most cases) when there is a problem . . . but it takes time. Older physicians have learned that the Tincture of Time is often the best course of treatment to follow.

Antibiotics require a certain period of time before they begin exerting their positive effects on the body. All too often I've heard patients complain that they don't feel any better after taking an antibiotic for only twenty-four or forty-eight hours. They then call their doctor complaining they aren't feeling better and want a different antibiotic. They don't realize that they didn't get sick in one day, and they're not going to get better in one day. The wise physician will reassure the patient, warn him of possible complicating signs and symptoms, and ask him to wait another day or so before making any changes. Unfortunately, our society has become one of instant gratification. We don't like to wait for anything. We want it now, and that includes getting better when we are ill. Patience is not a virtue that many of us possess.

Before about seventy-five years ago, the Tincture of Time was about all that we physicians could offer our patients. Modern medicines such as antibiotics and cardiac medicines just didn't exist. Doctors could use the occasional leech for bloodletting, apply a salve to a wound and, in dire circumstances, operate. (That often was enough to kill the healthiest patient.) Patience was a virtue that all physicians had to learn, and something that patients today must learn as well.

Detectives need facts to solve crimes. Physicians need facts to make an accurate diagnosis and they can only come from one place: from the patient. Here are some tips to help your patients make you a better doctor-detective:

10 Tips to Help Your Doctor Make the Correct Diagnosis

1. **Think about your problem before seeing your doctor and write down all the pertinent facts so you don't forget the most important things.**

2. **Decide what the key issues are that you want answered and prioritize them.**

3. **Think about your symptoms—when did they begin, how long do they last and what changes them for better or worse.**

4. **Tell your story succinctly so that your doctor can ask questions to clarify your concerns.**

5. **Don't be afraid to tell your doctor about the signs and symptoms that are bothering you even if he doesn't specifically ask about them.**

6. **Do mention anything that is different about you since your last visit because the change could be related to your medical problem or to a medicine you are taking.**

7. List all the medications and supplements you are taking.
8. Be honest about the level of pain that occurs during the physical examination. Downplaying this may cause the doctor to underestimate your problem.
9. Don't wait until the doctor is leaving the room before mentioning a particular concern you have or the problem might not get the attention it deserves.
10. Be sure to tell your doctor if you've had something like this previously or what you think your problem may be. (Patients are often right.)

5

Surgeons and the Art of Medicine

"The science of medicine is human biology and the art of medicine is everything else physicians do for their patients."

–Dr. Curt Tribble

Three surgeons are sitting in the surgical lounge discussing their cases for the morning.

Surgeon 1: "I'm glad my patient is a librarian. His organs will be in alphabetical order."

Surgeon 2: "How nice that my patient is a mathematician. All his organs will be numbered and I just put the numbers in order."

Surgeon 3: "Ha! Mine's the easiest case and the fastest. My patient is a politician: gutless, spineless and heartless."

The Student was extremely nervous as he entered the surgical scrub area with Jim Hamilton, the second-year resident. Jim was his teacher for that day on the cardiothoracic surgical rotation. It was his second day on surgery and his first time to actually see a surgical procedure. He had heard the stories about surgeons' personalities and tempers as they operated and now he was going to experience it first-hand. He wasn't sure what was going to be expected of him, and that made him even more nervous.

So far, surgery had been nothing like he expected. On the first day of his surgical rotation, Dr. Curt Tribble, the Chief of Thoracic Surgery, had oriented the twenty-four students on the various surgical rotations as to what would be expected of them. Dr. Tribble had taken him completely by surprise because he hadn't fit the Student's preconceived notion of surgeons. Dr. Tribble and Dr. Newburg, the co-leader of the students' surgical rotation, had led all the students through a discussion on why they had entered medicine.

They had also talked about goals and performance and explored subjects as different as what separated peak performing athletes, musicians and artists from the average. It seemed to have nothing to do with surgery but more to do with themselves and their own motivations. It seemed a little touchy-feely at first but the Student had to admit he enjoyed hearing his classmates' stories about how they had come to enter medical school. Many of the stories had surprised him. It seemed that so many of his classmates had been influenced in their choice to enter medical school by doctors they had known when they were young. He had not been ready to share his road to medicine because he didn't like that "group grope" kind of sharing. It was just too personal for him.

The Student's daydreaming was interrupted by the resident who handed him a surgical mask, told him to put it on and to begin the surgical scrub process. "Take this brush impregnated with antiseptic, wet your hands and arms and begin scrubbing for at least five minutes. This kills the bacteria on your skin and cuts down on the risk of infection for the patient. When you're done, come into the operating room and we'll begin scrubbing and draping the patient. By then, the rest of the team will be here and we can begin."

The Student began scrubbing furiously when he heard a

familiar voice behind him. "Student, didn't know you'd be here today. Are you on surgery now?"

Unbelievably, it was his Advisor. He couldn't escape him. He seemed to be everywhere. "Yes, sir, it's my first real day on surgery. The team that I'm on is about to do a triple vessel bypass on a man whose coronaries aren't too good."

"Who's doing the surgery?"

"It's Dr. Tribble. Do you know him very well?"

The Advisor laughed. "I sure do. He used to be one of my residents, and was one of the best. In fact, he was voted the Teacher of the Year by this year's medical school graduating class. He's won numerous teaching awards and is revered by his residents. You're really fortunate to be on his team. He'll be a great role model for you because he's a surgeon who's extremely well skilled in the Art of Medicine. If you get the chance, ask him what he does with each of his patients before they undergo bypass surgery."

With that, the Advisor turned off the water, put his hands into the air and pushed in the door to the adjacent operating room and left the Student to finish getting scrubbed. When the Student was done, he pushed through the opposite operating room door, mimicking his Advisor's motions. The patient was draped by the time the Student finished gowning. Dr. Hamilton showed him how to gown and then began the ritual of scrubbing the patient while instructing the Student in the finer details of prepping the patient. "Wound infections can be devastating to surgeons and can destroy all the hard work that they may have done inside the body. A good surgical prep can help prevent the majority of infections so this is no place to take short cuts."

The prep was almost complete when Dr. Tribble and his chief resident entered the operating room. They gowned while they again looked at the coronary angiograms. Dr. Tribble turned and said to the circulating nurse, "Time to start the music."

The Student wondered what that was all about until he saw the nurse go to a small CD player in the corner and put on a CD containing classic rock hits from the '70s. The chief resident waited until the music was on before officially beginning the surgery with a big midline incision of the patient's chest. Dr. Hamilton leaned toward the Student and whispered, "It's an old tradition with Dr. Tribble and many other surgeons to play music when they operate. The Boss loves the old rock classics."

Dr. Tribble turned to the Student and said, "Welcome to the most exciting surgery in medicine. You're now part of the greatest surgical team in the medical center. One key bit of advice for you while you're on our service . . . and for that matter, all others. The only dumb question is the one that's not asked. So, let's hear what's on your mind. What's your first question of the day?"

Why am I always on the spot? He's just like my Advisor. I'm the new guy on the block and know nothing, so why is he asking me anything? How can I not seem stupid with my first question?

The Student hesitated and almost stammered as he spoke, "I just saw my Advisor and he suggested that I ask you what you do with your patients before surgery. Do you tell them all about the procedure and what you're going to do?"

With his mask on, no one could see the huge smile on Dr. Tribble's face, but everyone could see it in his eyes. "So you've got the old guy too. You know, he was my Advisor in medical school as well, and he's been my mentor ever since."

Dr. Tribble looked back into the wound and called, "Clamp." He then clamped off a small bleeding artery that the resident then cauterized.

"Patients undergoing bypass surgery are generally scared to death . . . no pun intended. They all expect me to come talk to them about what we're going to do to them in the OR . . . all the technical stuff. What I've found is that they really don't want to know about it any more than they want to know how an airline pilot sets his computers or plots his course across the country. They want to have confidence that I'm well trained and that I'm skilled at what I do . . . even in emergencies. Student, here's the take-home message for you. Almost all of our patients desperately want permission to quit thinking about what we're going to do in here. They don't think they have permission to do that. What I ask them is, 'What gives meaning to your life? What gives you peace and happiness? What one thing helps you escape and recharges your batteries?' I hear millions of things from the people I ask. They NEVER fail to have an answer and it's often the simplest of things that give meaning to their lives. It's the desire to play with their grandchildren, to walk on the beach again or maybe to sit on the porch watching a sunset with their loved ones again."

Dr. Tribble then told the operating team that it would only be a few minutes before they were ready to put the patient on the cardiac perfusion machine. Once that was done, the team would begin sewing the grafts taken from the patient's legs around the blockages in the coronary arteries. He then turned to Dr. Hamilton. "Jim, where does today's patient find meaning in his life?"

"Boss, he loves to go fishing. He loves to get in his boat, float out on the lake near his house and get away from it all. It gives him time to think. He finds that he returns in a positive mood and appreciating all the blessings he has in his life. Those are his own words . . . not mine."

"Great, Jim. You've obviously spent some time with our friend here."

Dr. Tribble interrupted his story briefly to tell the team they were one minute away from placing the patient on the bypass pump. He continued his story without missing a beat . . . a good thing for a cardiac surgeon. He then continued, "Once I know what the real joys are in their life, I tell them, 'I'm going to do this operation to make you well

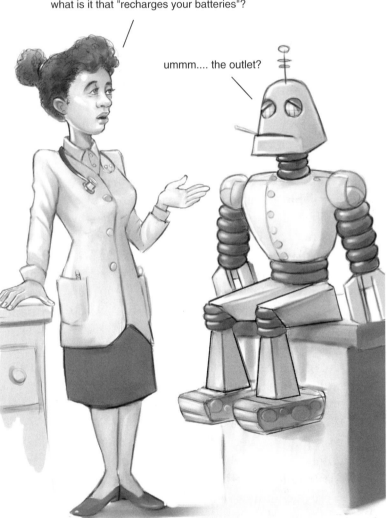

again. Here's your part of the deal. I don't want you to think about your operation. I want you to think about going fishing, in the case of our patient today. I want you to picture it in your mind. I want you to think about being there. To imagine how it feels, the smells and the air. Don't think about what we're going to be doing. You don't need to worry about any of what we do. You've got one job and that's to look ahead. Look ahead to where you want to be. If you look at your feet, you'll fail but if you look at the horizon, you'll get to your goal.

"Then, I make them promise to send me letters with pictures of them doing what they like the most. And you know, each week, I get letters from at least one of our patients. This is what makes it all worthwhile to me. This is what energizes me as a doctor. This is what Dr. Newburg is talking about when he talks about following your dream."

At that point, all talking stopped except for that related to the surgical task at hand. The operation proceeded without problem and in relative quiet. This was fine with the Student because it gave him time to think about what Dr. Tribble had said.

This is all so different from what I expected. It isn't just about cracking someone's chest. They actually connect with their patients. I can feel the excitement in the room when Dr. Tribble's talking. It's almost contagious and most of the residents on this service seem to be the same way.

As Dr. Tribble was closing the chest, he began to tell his team about an incident that had taken place with his mechanic the day before. "My car needed some work on the valves. When I brought it in, my mechanic was busy working on another car. He saw me and asked if he could ask a question. I of course told him, 'No problem.' Here was his question to me: 'So Doc, look at this engine. I also open up the heart of the engine, take out valves, fix 'em, put in new parts and when I finish, this will work just like a new one.

My question is so how come I get such a pittance and you get the really big bucks, when you and I are doing basically the same work?' You know what I told him?"

No one had any idea so Dr. Tribble continued with the story; "I smiled and just told him, 'Try doing it with the engine running like I do.'" The whole operating room burst into laughter because they all knew what he said was so true. When you had someone's life in your hands, the risk was higher . . . and so should be the reward.

At the end of almost three hours, the chief resident finished closing the patient's chest while Dr. Tribble watched and, when done, signaled the end to another successful surgery. Now, it was mainly up to the patient to do the slow work of healing and the really hard job of rehabilitating himself, and making changes in his lifestyle to reduce his risk of future cardiac problems. It was to be the final surgery of the day for the cardiothoracic team before going to surgery clinic. There they would evaluate new patients for surgery and recheck patients who had undergone bypass surgery previously. It was a long, grueling day but rewarding when one could hear and see the success enjoyed by the returning patients.

Dr. Tribble started to leave the OR when he suddenly stopped and said, "Student, I almost forgot something that I like to give to every new person on our service. It's an excellent article written by Dr. Francis Moore that provides a wonderful philosophy on surgery. It's got some real pearls of wisdom in it that I expect all my surgeons to know and to follow. I've got a meeting with the residents in the morning so maybe we can discuss it after that. See you then."

The rest of the day was uneventful but extremely busy. The Student had no problem sleeping that night but it seemed like he'd only been asleep briefly when the alarm sounded the next morning at 5:00 AM.

Why do surgeons insist on getting started so darn early? It's sure a mystery to me and another reason I'm becoming a radiologist.

The Student arrived in time to review the lab work and pre-op data for that morning's patients with two of the residents. It had been checked previously but it never hurt to recheck things, especially since charts could be misplaced and data put with the wrong patient. They also went over the previous night's admissions to make sure they would be ready for presentation on morning rounds. The rest of the team arrived by 6:15 AM and rounds got underway.

The Attending for the month was Dr. Jim Maher, also known by all the residents as "The Cookie Monster." Dr. Maher was a big, gentle man with a huge heart and a waistline to match. He had never had a meal, or a dessert, that he didn't like—and his waistline was definitely a testament to that fact. He believed that surgery should as fun as possible, since there was already enough stress associated with most operations. You were operating on very sick people who could possibly die so a little comic relief would go a long way to relieving the tension associated with it. It was always amazing to anyone who saw him operate that a man with such huge hands could have such a delicate surgical touch. He was famous on the surgery service for the many medical aphorisms that all the residents liked to repeat.

On this particular day, one of the braver residents was out in front of the surgical team doing his best imitation of Dr. Maher. He had stuffed a pillow under his surgical scrub shirt and was walking around while moving his arms wildly and repeating all the little surgical aphorisms that Dr. Maher was famous for among the housestaff. "Never let the skin stand between you and the diagnosis. Nice people get bad diseases. Stool does not clot. A chance to cut is a chance to cure, and it's always a chance to cut. The pancreas is in the back of the abdomen so no one messes with it."

Unfortunately, and unseen by the budding young actor-resident, Dr. Maher walked up behind him and yelled in the gruffest voice possible, "Dr. Fox, you've heard the old saying that you can't make chicken salad out of chicken manure. Well, that's what I'm trying to do with you when I try to turn you into a surgeon. You didn't do a bad imitation but you forgot my favorite, 'If you can't run with the big dogs, stay on the porch.' I'm the biggest dog on surgery and you had better stay on the porch until you're ready." Then, Dr. Maher turned to the rest of the team and laughed heartily. "Now, let's go to surgery, do some cutting, and have some fun."

The rest of the group headed off to surgery while the Student left the group to meet with Dr. Tribble and the twenty-three other students on the surgical service. It was a point of pride within the surgical group that the education of medical students was not left to junior faculty or residents but was taught in great part by the senior faculty. Who better to mentor the young people and who better to serve as role models for those in their formative years?

Dr. Tribble always dressed extremely well and had the lean athletic body to carry it off. He not only tried to set an example for his residents and staff in the OR but also in his personal life. He spent many hours with his wife and children and also found time to exercise to keep himself as fit as possible. Surgery was hard work and you had to be in shape to maintain your edge.

"Welcome to the surgical service again, students. I guarantee you that this will be one of the best rotations you will have while in medical school. You'll learn how to take care of sick patients. You'll learn some basic surgical skills that you can use anywhere, and hopefully, you'll learn an approach to medicine that will serve you well for the rest of your life. Ours is different from many other services, but it's one that seems to serve our patients best.

"I'm now going to hand out a book on surgery provided by the Ethicon Company, one of our suppliers of surgical suture. It's an excellent book that teaches you the basics of wound healing, the differences in suture materials and when to use them, how to tie various surgical knots and, finally, some tips on how to suture different types of wounds. I expect you to read it and know the sections on wound healing and what one should think about when closing different types of wounds. We'll reinforce and expand on all this but we expect you to know the basics.

"For those of you with an appreciation for history, you'll see that we've come a long way in our understanding of wound healing. Up until the nineteenth century it was believed that wounds did not heal well unless they contained what was known as 'laudable pus.' It took Lister and others to teach us that the use of antiseptics would enable our wounds to remain clean and heal faster. His work saved untold thousands of lives but it wasn't without risk to his personal reputation. He had to go against the grain of commonly held knowledge and it came at a great personal cost to him. It was only with scientific fact that he was able to change the thinking of others. It's one of the reasons we require our residents to do a year of research prior to becoming a surgeon. We want them to advance our knowledge of science but more importantly, they need to learn what constitutes good research so that they can evaluate what's presented in the scientific literature. To reinforce that point, does anyone know what percentage of peer reviewed articles in respectable medical journals had major scientific flaws contained in them?"

The silence in the room was almost unnerving. No one wanted to be wrong and show his or her ignorance, especially since this was the chief of surgery asking the question.

Dr. Tribble laughed, "O.K., we're going to play 'Who Wants to Be a Millionaire.' Your choices for $250,000 are 20%, 40%, 60% or 80% of the articles contained in good medical journals have major scientific flaws."

A brave soul in the middle of the room put up his hand. "Twenty percent?"

"Pretty close, Dr. Baum. It's 40% but you get $10,000 in goodwill as a consolation prize for being the only student brave enough to play."

Everyone laughed along with Dr. Tribble, who then got up and paced around the front of the room as he talked. "This statistic should be extremely unnerving to you all. Scientific research is put in print and yet contains data that are misleading, that lack scientific credibility and that even lead people to draw false conclusions. My point to all of you is that you need to be careful about what you read and how you interpret it. There are excellent books that will help you to understand the medical literature and I strongly suggest you read them and learn the key points. Remember what the British politician, Benjamin Disraeli, once said, 'There are lies, damned lies and statistics.' You can use data to support your argument but what's really important is to present the data fairly and objectively."

One of the students in the back had her hand raised. "Yes, Dr. Benson, you have a question?"

"Yes, sir, what are some of the things that you think are important for us to learn while we're on the surgery rotation and how do we go about it?"

"Good question. There are some definite things that I want you to learn and much of that can be found in the article by Dr. Moore that all of you should have received. One of the other things we have found that will help you get the most out of your time with us in surgery is to have you keep a notebook, a personalized journal of your experience while here on surgery. This is entirely up to you but," and here he paused dramatically, "you will receive extra credit if it's completed." The entire group laughed at this last comment because every medical student was always concerned about his or her grades.

"We want you to compile a list of the patients you see, and what you learn from each. Then, we want you to add to the notebook any articles that you find useful pertaining to that particular case. You can paste in the chapters from your surgical textbook as well because they don't do you any good unless you read them in a context you can relate to and remember. This is step number one.

"In a nutshell, what we hope you will learn is how to evaluate patients who have a possible surgical problem, when they are physiologically prepared enough so that it's safe to operate on them, and how to care for them following surgery. Caring for patients after surgery involves a lot more than healing their surgical incisions. It often involves healing their psyche as well. We know in cardiothoracic surgery that we can perform a beautiful, successful coronary bypass surgical procedure but unless we rehabilitate the patient psychologically as well as physically, we still may have a 'cardiac cripple.' Some surgeons are excellent technicians and operate beautifully, but that's not all it takes to be a good surgeon. The best surgeons know that there is an 'Art' to Medicine as well. Your patient must believe in you and trust you; only then will he become a partner in the total healing process that occurs after the actual surgical healing has taken place."

From the back of the room a female voice interrupted Dr. Tribble. "Curt, can I say something to reinforce that last point with our students?"

"Sure, Mary, your input's always welcome. Ladies and gentleman, this is Dr. Mary Hammond. She's one of our Ob-Gyn surgeons who's won many teaching awards."

"Dr. Tribble's last point is so important and, unfortunately, is overlooked by many surgeons. A perfect example of this involves women with breast cancer. A surgeon can do a beautiful job of actually removing all of the cancer that can be identified but that's just the beginning of the healing process. If a woman has had a mastectomy, just think of the tremendous psychological trauma to her body image. How does she overcome that initial feeling of disfigurement and unattractiveness? How does she deal with the fear of her cancer recurring or the fear that eats at her every time she goes in for a checkup or another mammogram? How does she get on with her life when she feels like she's been sucker-punched by the Big C? Have you identified the most competent oncologists and radiation experts to provide the additional therapy that she will need? That woman is going to be looking to you to point her toward the resources she'll need to recover on many different levels. You obviously can't provide all the services yourself but you do need to know where your patient can get the support she needs. It can be patient support groups, community resources, counselors, the Internet or a combination of many things."

"Thanks, Mary, that's a perfect example of why good medicine requires physicians who are skilled in both the Art and the Science of medicine. The final clinical skill or bit of diagnostic acumen that I'd like to see you and all my residents acquire constitutes what I call the '**Diagnostic Imperatives.**' The Diagnostic Imperatives, or DIs, are those diagnoses or problems that are so important to a patient's health that if you miss them, the patient has an increased chance of dying."

"Well, what are these diagnoses and how do we recognize them?" asked Dr. Stenger again.

Dr. Tribble smiled before replying, "I'll list some of the conditions and tell you a little about them but part of what you'll need to research, learn, and put in your notebooks while here on surgery is how to recognize and diagnose them. I can't emphasize it enough. You always have to consider them as part of your differential diagnoses. If you don't, then you'll never make the correct diagnosis. These DIs aren't easy to recognize because they can mimic other conditions that are less life threatening and much more common. It's easy to think of the common things but not so easy to think of the rarer problems that can kill a patient if missed."

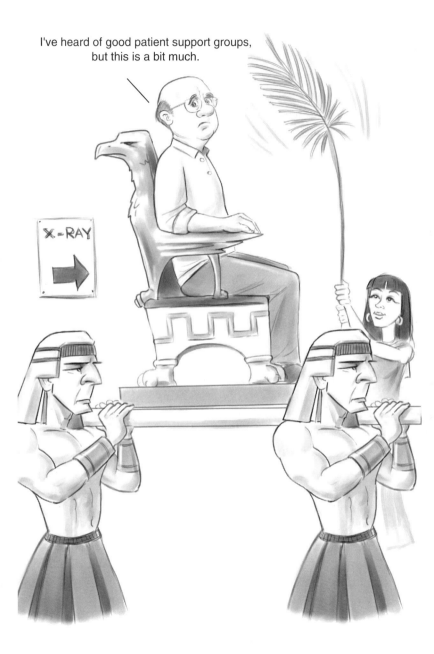

Dr. Tribble placed a slide on the overhead projector and began to explain each point.

1. **Acute appendicitis**—infection or inflammation of the appendix. Can rupture and cause peritonitis of the abdomen. Mimics PID, ectopic pregnancy, bowel obstruction, irritable bowel disease or simple constipation.
2. **Aortic aneurysm**—a ballooning of the wall of the aorta that can lead to rupture and a massive internal bleed. Mimics abdominal pain, heart attack and back pain.
3. **Bacterial meningitis**—a bacterial infection of the lining of the brain. Mimics headache, sinus infection and upper respiratory infection. High index of suspicion needed. Even with early treatment, can result in residual brain damage.
4. **Ectopic pregnancy**—a pregnancy that occurs and begins to grow in the Fallopian tubes rather than in the uterus. It can mimic appendicitis, kidney stone, urinary tract infection, pelvic inflammatory disease (PID), abdominal pain or bowel obstruction, to mention a few.
5. **Epiglottitis**—a serious infection of the epiglottis found almost exclusively in young children. Mimics upper respiratory infections, strep throat, tonsillitis and croup. Touch the epiglottis and the patient's throat can close, requiring an emergency tracheotomy so he can breathe.
6. **Meningococcemia**—a bacterial infection of the blood that may simply look like a fever and a rash. Mimics many viral infections except for the characteristic rash.
7. **Myocardial infarction**—the classic heart attack caused by the blockage of the coronary arteries in the heart. Early treatment can reverse or prevent further damage to the heart or death. Mimics esophageal problems, heartburn, shoulder pain or jaw pain.
8. **Stroke**—blockage/infarction or hemorrhage of the brain. Mimics headache, transient ischemic attacks (TIA) or

meningitis. Early treatment can reverse symptoms in many cases.

9. **Testicular torsion**—a twisting of the testicle internally so that the blood supply is compromised. If not corrected, the testicle will be lost. Can be confused with epididymitis, localized cellulitis and sometimes a hernia.

"Like the 7 deadly sins, these DIs, if missed, can cause unnecessary death or severe disability. Always consider them in your differential diagnosis and you'll never go wrong. Any questions? "

Another of the female students quickly raised her hand. "Some of the problems you have listed aren't really surgical problems. Why should we be concerned about these on the surgery service?"

"Another good question. Here's my take on that one. Some DIs are clearly not surgical issues but you may be consulted because some of the conditions or diagnoses that they mimic are surgical in nature. You may be the only person who thinks of the correct diagnosis, so it just might give you the opportunity to save someone's life. Plus, you never know what situation you might find yourself in medically so you'd better learn these things. Let's say you're off volunteering somewhere and you're asked to do something more than just straight surgery. Knowing these things will keep you and your patient out of trouble."

Dr. Tribble again began to pace across the front of the room while he spoke. It was a habit they would all come to associate with him as he spoke to groups, no matter how big or small. "Let me share a couple of war stories with you that will illustrate my point. The first involved a young lady in her twenties who came to the ER complaining of right-sided abdominal pain. The first-year resident on duty thought it was appendicitis because the woman had a low-grade fever, was nauseated, had a slightly elevated white blood count and was tender when touched on the right side. The surgical resident was called and they decided that the young lady needed to have her appendix removed so they began to prepare the patient for surgery. One of the female students on the surgical rotation who had heard this same talk, just like you, noticed that no pregnancy test had been done. She spoke to one of the other residents who agreed to order one. It came back positive. Suddenly, everything had changed. An ultrasound of the abdomen was done which showed an ectopic pregnancy. The woman did go to surgery but for an entirely different reason. A possible surgical disaster was averted thanks to the heads-up thinking of a medical student. I personally was pleased from two perspectives. First, it was a student who used her head and wasn't afraid to speak up. Second, the resident she spoke to was open enough to really listen to a suggestion from a student.

"The second case involved an older gentleman who came to the ER in the middle of the night, complaining of abdominal pain. He was in significant pain and mentioned that he hadn't had a bowel movement in three days. The plain films of his abdomen showed lots of stool in his bowel but not much else could be seen. All his lab tests were negative. The ER doctor thought it was probably a case of simple constipation but he couldn't entirely rule out a bowel obstruction so he asked for a surgical consult. At about 2 a.m., the second-year surgical resident saw the patient and, despite the hour, took another history from the patient. He let the patient tell his story and heard the patient say that he felt a tearing sensation inside when his pain began. He also felt some pain in his back. The resident's antenna went up immediately. Patients with acute dissecting aortic aneurysms often describe their condition in this way. The resident then got a special CT scan and made the correct diagnosis. If you fail to make this diagnosis and treat patients for some other problem like constipation, they often dissect further and eventually rupture at the site of the aneurysm. Fortunately, the patient underwent emergency surgery for his aneurysm and he had no further problems.

"Unfortunately, our morbidity and mortality conferences always remind us of those cases that don't turn out with happy endings. As is the case with the other parts of our lives, it's our mistakes that teach us the lessons that have the greatest impact and stay with us the longest. Any other questions?"

None of the students had questions, so Dr. Tribble dismissed the group. They all had plenty to do and so much to learn.

✤ *Perspectives for Doctors* ✤

Two of the best teachers of both the Art and Science of surgery that I personally know are Dr. James Patrick O'Leary, the head of surgery at the Louisiana State University (LSU) School of Medicine, and Dr. Curt Tribble, chief of cardiothoracic surgery at the University of Virginia. Each is very deeply involved in the education of residents and students and believes strongly that you must model what you want the end result to be. They also possess two characteristics that all good teachers must have—a joy of learning and a great curiosity about people and life. They constantly look at medicine and life and ask "Why?" These two surgeons believe that how they train their residents will have an impact on doctors, and patients, for many generations to come. These young people will be the teachers of tomorrow and you can't teach others what you don't know.

The teaching of surgeons raises one big question. Is it important to see a surgeon who specializes in certain surgeries or is a general surgeon acceptable for all surgeries? In some cases, it makes a tremendous difference. A couple of recent studies address that point directly. A 2001 study in the *Journal of Vascular Surgery* demonstrated significantly lower mortality rates in patients who have abdominal aortic aneurysms repaired by vascular or cardiac surgeons than by general surgeons. Two other studies, one in Canada and the other in Australia, confirm that board certified colorectal surgeons had significantly lower death rates and complication rates when compared to other hospital surgeons. Training does make a significant difference. The key question patients should ask is, "If you needed the same surgery I did, who would you get to do your surgery?" That is always telling. Remember it just may be someone's life that's at stake.

These exact relationships are also true for trauma care. Optimal outcomes can be achieved at greatest efficiency if care is restricted to relatively few dedicated trauma centers. Why is this so? The belief is that higher patient volumes will lead to greater experience and that this experience translates into better patient outcomes. Study results strongly support this premise because mortality and length of stay are greatly improved when trauma case volumes exceed 650 cases per year, but only in those patients at high risk for adverse outcomes.

Many people are careful about picking their surgeon but they also need to learn more about the person who is putting them to sleep. In some operations the anesthesiologist might just be the most important person in the operating room. A recent NBC report on the NBC Nightly News highlighted this very issue. Fortunately, anesthesiology is likely the premier medical specialty in addressing issues of patient safety. Why? First, the specialty of anesthesiology had strong leaders who were willing to admit that patient safety was not all that it could be and to look for solutions. Second, the cost of malpractice insurance was becoming astronomical for anesthesiologists in the United States and many knew that patient safety had to be improved if this were to improve.

This marked improvement in patient safety in the last thirty-five years came about by using a number of strategies that can be used elsewhere in medicine. Here's how they did it:

1. **Applying technological solutions to clinical problems**— By using electrocardiography to measure heart rhythms, pulse oximetry to measure oxygen and capnography to measure carbon dioxide levels, they are constantly monitoring patients to detect problems early.
2. **Use of practice parameters**—Standards and guidelines were adopted in the 1980s to provide guidance and direction for the diagnosis, management and treatment of specific clinical problems. The first set of standards was on basic monitoring.
3. **Applying the systems approach to safety**—Anesthesia pioneered work on analyses of the processes within the specialty as well as designing systems to reduce the chance of human error.
4. **Utilizing patient simulators**—Anesthesiologists pioneered the development of computer screen and mannequin-based interactive patient simulators for training at all levels.

Much remains to be done. There are still many gaps in patient safety to be addressed. Patient simulators exist in only a few facilities and so are available to only a small fraction of anesthesiologists and anesthetists. Clinicians still practice even though they are unable to perform optimally due to fatigue, illness or stress. Basic standards are not always followed. Finally, the specialty is not unique in failing to require continuing skills training or performance assessments as part of their ongoing certification.

Surgery itself is not without risk even in the best of hands. There are definite risks from being put to sleep, from just being in the hospital, from adverse reactions tomedicines, or from some unforeseen complication of the surgery itself. Even the simplest procedures can have unforeseen complications. There was a report recently about an eight-year-old boy who died from a postoperative hemorrhage after a routine tonsillectomy. Bad things do happen despite everyone's best efforts. Often, patients take these things so much for granted that they really don't pay attention to or don't understand what the surgeon has said about the risks (and they often freely sign the consent form) or the surgeon views the procedure as so routine that he or she fails to mention some of the more severe complications because they may never have had any of them. Patients need to think carefully before undergoing surgery.

Here are a few questions that all patients (doctors can be patients also, and should consider these questions for their patients as well) should consider:

10 Questions to Ask Your Surgeon Before Surgery

1. What can I do before surgery to make myself ready and increase my chances for success?
2. Which hospital has the team best skilled in this type of procedure?
3. How many procedures has my surgeon done of this type of surgery?
4. What are the most common complications associated with this surgery?
5. What medicines should I stop before surgery and when should I stop them?
6. What are my choices for anesthesia for this surgery? What are the pros and cons of each?
7. Where can I go to obtain more information about the procedure and my alternatives?
8. Should I get a second opinion?
9. What are the risks of delaying surgery or trying a non-surgical approach to treatment before surgery?
10. If your doctor were having this surgery, whom would he get to do the operation?

6

Liberal Arts and Renaissance Men . . . and Women

"Commonplaces never become tiresome. It is we who become tired when we cease to be curious and appreciative . . . (We) find that it is not a new scene which is needed, but a new viewpoint."

–Norman Rockwell

". . . it is habits of mind and standards of performance that we should aspire to teach and not the illusion of enduring facts."

–J. Bishop

The main campus of the university was beautiful. It was landscaped with many different types of flowering plants and shrubs as well as plenty of large mature trees, such as oaks and maples of various kinds to provide shade in the hot summer months. Fall had arrived and brought a beautiful warm day with hardly a cloud in the sky. It was one of those great days that made you glad to be alive. The Student was pleased that the Advisor had asked him to walk with him to the library on the main campus, since it gave him the chance to be outside and enjoy the fabulous weather

"Well, Student, what have you been up to these last couple of weeks?" the Advisor asked. "Aren't you on the cardiology service now? How do you like it?"

The Student wondered what to say to his Advisor because his medical rotation on cardiology wasn't going as well as he'd hoped. There was so much to learn, and he was having the hardest time differentiating between the various heart sounds. At times, the murmurs all sounded the same. It was discouraging to say the least. The one good thing about this rotation was all the work with ultrasound imaging and PET scans. The radiology part was the most exciting to him. Maybe he'd share those thoughts, but certainly not his feelings of incompetence.

"Cardiology is OK. What I'm really enjoying is all the radiological testing we get to do on our patients. What did you ever do before you had all this imaging technology? I can't imagine not having CT scans, MRIs or ultrasounds to evaluate patients."

The Advisor smiled before replying, "I know the days when we didn't have all our present medical technology must seem like the Dark Ages to you. You probably compare all these new diagnostic toys as a period of enlightenment much like the Renaissance was to the Middle Ages. Hey, since I brought up the Middle Ages, what discovery or invention of that time do you think had the greatest impact on the people and culture of that period . . . and maybe today as well?"

The Student looked at the Advisor with a dazed look on his face. *The Renaissance and the Middle Ages? Where did he pull those things from? I thought that we were talking about cardiology. Simply amazing! The next thing he's going to be off on will be King Arthur and the Knights of the Round Table. I'm not even sure when the Middle Ages were. I thought it occurred when people were be-*

tween thirty-five and fifty-five. Discoveries? Inventions? There was nothing of great importance that came out of science then. The real scientific advances have only occurred recently. Where does he get this stuff? Jeez, why did I ever agree to go for a walk with him today?

"Was it machines of war?"

"Uh . . . not quite, but I do agree they've had quite an impact on people today. Have you ever heard of someone by the name of Gutenberg?"

"Yeah, of course, but I learned about him in grade school, and frankly, he just didn't come to mind."

"Unbelievable! Let me ask you, did you have any history or review of civilization courses as part of your college education?"

"No, sir, I was a science major and didn't need any of that stuff to get into medical school. My college advisor didn't suggest them, and I certainly didn't see a need for them either. What good would they do me as a doctor? The medical schools like science majors and they really don't ask about all that liberal arts junk."

The Advisor sighed sadly. "Unfortunately, you're right when it comes to what medical schools look for in most cases. They look at MCAT scores and GPAs as a screen and don't get much further many times . . . but that's a whole different story. I admit that I do have a bias for wanting doctors to have a decent background in the liberal arts, but I'm also the first to admit that we certainly need a mixture of students to meet the different demands within medicine.

"Well, Student, here's the answer to my question, and a little history lesson for you. Gutenberg was a German who invented the printing press around 1564. Before his invention, whatever books existed had to be written by hand. Any copies of those books also had to be done by hand. This was so time-consuming and expensive that only the rich—the elite—had access to books. The masses were uneducated and would have remained that way if it weren't for

Gutenberg. With his invention, books for the first time became accessible to the common man. I'd say 'woman' but they really didn't believe in the education of women during those times. Knowledge, ideas, and literature became the domain of every person. No longer was there an excuse for being ignorant. Schools could have textbooks and ideas could be spread to the masses, even if unpopular to the ruling class. His invention would forever revolutionize society. To this day, we owe Gutenberg a tremendous debt. Just think where you'd be if you couldn't buy all the wonderful texts you could, but had to rely on word of mouth to spread the knowledge. Pretty scary, huh?"

Neither man said anything further until they reached the library. The sign in front advertised the special exhibition inside, "The Humanity of Man as Expressed in Art." The Student looked at the sign with some dismay.

Please don't tell me that he dragged me up here to look at a bunch of paintings. What has this got to do with medicine? Next thing you know, he'll be taking me to concerts, museums, or worse, ballet. Give me a good football or basketball game any time. I don't have time for this with all the science I've got to learn.

The Advisor opened the door of the library and ushered the Student inside. He walked them back to the exhibition area before speaking. "There are a couple of paintings that I'd especially like for you to see today. They'll tell you a great deal about our understanding of the human condition as expressed in art."

They moved past a few paintings before stopping in front of one that had a doctor dressed in 1900s-style clothing sitting beside the bed of a sick child. The parents were huddled together in obvious distress in the background. "This is a masterpiece on loan from the Tate Gallery in London and is called *The Doctor*. It was painted by Sir Luke Fildes and was inspired by the memory of Fildes' son. It's a powerful depiction of the compassion that a physician can bring to a

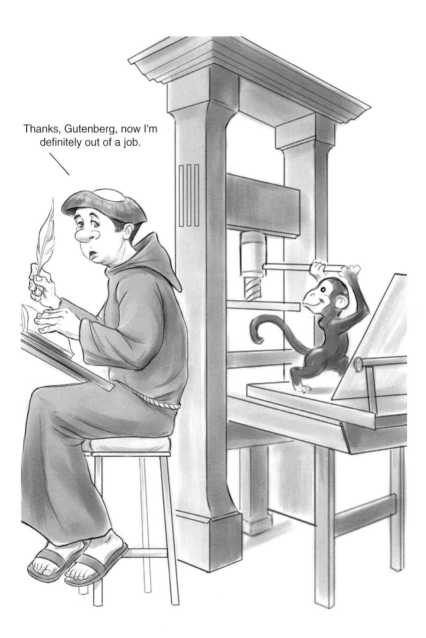

family, especially when there is nothing else that he has to offer in the way of treatment or aid. It had to be so terribly frustrating for the physicians of that era not to have much to offer their patients in the way of treatment. This painting so moves and inspires me that I have a copy of it in my office. It's a constant reminder for me that our patients need compassion, caring and someone to listen to them . . . as well as all the wonderful science we can now offer."

The Advisor then moved around the corner to an alcove containing a series of paintings done by Norman Rockwell. "Sit down here with me and look at these paintings for a moment while I explain Rockwell to you. For many people, Norman Rockwell was one of the greatest American painters ever. He told stories or narratives with paint that glorified ordinary Americans and imbued the people in his works with warmth, humility and humor. His works were too sentimental for many critics but were embraced by the average American. To get his picture on canvas, Rockwell had to listen to the story that all people have inside them. This is the same challenge that all physicians have. They have to find a way to get their patients to tell them the story of their lives. Without this, the doctor is treating only the symptoms, and not the total person."

The Student sat transfixed by the paintings in front of him. Rockwell's *The Four Freedoms* were the centerpieces of this part of the exhibition, and something in them clearly moved the future doctor. He had heard what his Advisor had said and could understand why Rockwell was so popular with most people. He seemed to capture the American spirit. In these pictures there was something that spoke to every man and woman. People could easily see a part of themselves in the people and stories he had depicted.

Why haven't I ever heard about these artists and their wonderful paintings before? How can my Advisor know so much about so many different subjects? He's the Chief of Surgery, so it doesn't leave him much time for anything else so when did he possibly learn about all this stuff?

At that point, the Advisor interrupted the Student's thoughts. "Got to run because I've got a young lady waiting for me back at the medical center."

The Student raised his eyebrows in surprise.

"No, it's nothing like that. It happens to be a young lady on whom I did a colon resection for Crohn's disease about three months ago. She wanted to see me to share some of her experiences trying to deal with her disease. She happens to be an artist and hopes to put together a book that would help other young people deal with the issues associated with having to defecate into a bag on their sides."

"Don't let me rush you. Feel free to stay here for as long as you want. Some of the history of these paintings you'll find quite remarkable. Oh, I almost forgot. Here's another article I brought for you to read that I'd like to discuss with you later. It's written by my friend, Dr. J. Patrick O'Leary, one of the leading educators in the field of surgery, and head of the surgical program at the LSU School of Medicine. He's mentored many students who now have gone on to be great teachers and leaders themselves. He's a great role model for us all. One of his strongest beliefs is that physicians need to view their medical school and residency as the start of their medical education. It's merely the first step in what should be lifelong learning. He also espouses a liberal arts education. It exposes people to a wide variety of thinking, and you'll soon find that all great thinkers had that in common. They had a great sense of curiosity about the world and the people around them, and they were constantly learning."

The Advisor turned, started to leave and then stopped. "Why don't you meet me in my office in about two hours? See you then."

The Advisor was at his desk when the Student returned.

"Come on in. Sit down and relax. Well, what did you think of Dr. O'Leary's paper?"

"It's nice but not my cup of tea. I'm still not sure all those liberal arts that you're so fond of are needed for me to be a good doctor."

The Advisor stretched his arms over his head, got up and started to pace around his office as he spoke. "The Greeks and the Romans believed that an educated man had to learn literature, philosophy and the arts before he was even allowed to undertake the study of the sciences. They felt that these studies provided not only a way to free the mind, but a means of understanding the human condition. Michael Eisner, the CEO of Walt Disney, was a double major in college. He studied both English and theater, and he believes it's an important reason for his success today." The Advisor walked over to his bookshelf and reached in to retrieve a book before continuing, "Here's something that Eisner's said that I think applies equally as well to medicine: 'Literature is unbelievably helpful, because no matter what business you are in, you are dealing with interpersonal relationships. It gives you an appreciation of what makes people tick.' There's nothing Mickey Mouse about that statement is there, Student?" laughed the Advisor. "What I'm trying to get across to you is that without the arts, the science doesn't mean as much. The same can be said for medicine today. Learning the Art of Medicine without learning the Science will spell failure for you as a doctor . . . and vice-versa; the Science without the Art makes you incomplete as a physician.

"Let me give you a practical example of how the liberal arts are used in the every day practice of medicine. You've seen how prescriptions are written and all the different abbreviations that are used. It may seem like gobbledy-gook but all these have a meaning that is derived from the Latin language. For instance, when we write "h.s." to indicate taking a prescription at bedtime, it's derived from the Latin *hora somni*—at the hour of sleep. When you write "t.i.d.," it stands for *tercem in die* or three times a day. Trust me, the liberal arts are alive and well in medicine today.

"You've told me that you're interested in old movies and that ultimately, you'd like to do something in that arena one day. To do things like this, you have to be able to write, to get in touch with those thoughts, ideas and emotions that flow through all men and women. These are the things that liberal arts bring to you. Look at some of the great physician writers and poets such as William Carlos Williams, Lewis Thomas, and Anton Chekhov, the great Russian writer. Student, do you know why I'm interested in the history of medicine?"

"Honestly, no, I can't imagine because none of that really interests me."

The Advisor laughed. "I can certainly understand where you're coming from because I used to be that way at one time in my life. What changed my way of thinking were two professors that I had in college. The first was Dr. Betty Baker. She was my biology teacher and intertwined history with her medical lectures. One of her favorite sayings was 'Those who fail to study history are doomed to repeat the mistakes of the past.' She'd then go on and share some historical story that would knock my socks off. I can tell you that I never expected to hear about history from a biology professor.

"The second professor who helped to create my love of history was Fr. Raphael Bridge. He taught one of those history of civilization courses required of all students at Belmont Abbey College. For the first time in my life I learned that there were political, economic, social and religious influences that shaped every major event in history. It was fascinating to see how all these things would come together and alter the course of history forever. For instance, do you know what one of the greatest influences on the formation of medical schools and hospitals was?"

The Student again got that glazed look on his face that the Advisor had quickly come to learn meant that he had no clue. The Student thought for a minute and hazarded a guess. "Was it Hippocrates?"

"Not a bad guess, since he's considered the father of medicine and was one of the earliest persons to make observations about how disease affects people. Actually, the Crusades were the event that had the greatest impact on the formation of hospitals and medical schools. Up until that time, there was only <u>one</u> real center of medical study, and that was at Salerno in Italy. The Crusades took place roughly around 1100 AD. When the Crusaders left and traveled across Europe to attack the infidels in the East, many were hurt in battle or got sick along the way. The only place to get medical care was back in their countries of origin so they had to be shipped back home for care. As a result, most died along the way and never made it back. To counter this, groups such as the Knights of the Hospitalers sprang up to help care for the sick and injured along the way. To this end, they formed hospitals in different cities along the route of the Crusades. It's fascinating isn't it? You're probably wondering how I manage to find time for learning all these different things? Am I right?"

The Student nodded his head up and down emphatically. "That exact thought crossed my mind when we were up in the library looking at those wonderful paintings."

"The answer's fairly simple to me. It's curiosity. My father and mother always encouraged my questions and then urged me to conduct experiments to get some of the answers. I never realized just how important curiosity was until I came across a book about the person who probably had the brightest mind in all history. The book was entitled *How to Think Like Leonardo da Vinci—Seven Steps to Genius Every Day.* Leonardo knew the importance of continuous learning 'Just as iron rusts from disuse, and stagnant water putrefies, or when cold turns to ice, so our intellect wanes unless it's kept in use.' In the book the author states that 'an insatiable, curious approach to life and an unrelenting quest for continuous learning' are what every great mind possesses. What I've found is that these attributes are also what make life fun and interesting for me. You can always find excuses why not to start learning but it's really never too late, no matter what your age."

"It's as simple as that?" asked the Student.

"I believe it is. There are many people who serve as classic examples of all this. Look at Grandma Moses who took up painting at such a ripe old age and became so famous. Look at the person at 3M who discovered Post-it Notes. All discoveries started with the basic question, 'What if?' Just think about your own experience as a filmmaker. If you didn't look at things in a different way and ask What, How, When, or Why, you wouldn't try anything new or different. That's how breakthroughs really occur.

"To help get you started, I took the liberty of getting you a copy of *How to Think Like Leonardo da Vinci.* Now the rest is up to you.

"Sorry," the Advisor said with a laugh, "but I've got to run. I've got a tennis lesson, so see you next week."

The Advisor dashed off as the Student sat in the chair and slowly started to read.

✧ *Perspectives for Doctors* ✧

With all the emphasis on business and technology today, a liberal arts education may seem like something that's a throwback to an earlier era. In fact, if one looks at the CEOs of the United States' 1000 largest companies as the executive search firm Spencer Stuart did, you will quickly see that only one-third of these CEOs have a master of business administration degree, while the rest have a variety of degrees with most majoring in liberal arts. The CEOs interviewed for that survey said the liberal arts help them to think "out of the box," to wrestle with ethical dilemmas and to approach problems in a systematic, orderly fashion. What greater set of skills could young physicians want as they approach the demands of medical practice today?

Dr. James Patrick O'Leary is currently the interim dean at the LSU Medical Center in New Orleans. Not only is he a surgeon but also an artist, an athlete, a preservationist of history and a committed family man. He has been the president of numerous national and specialty medical organizations and is a leader in the area of surgical education. He promotes the ongoing continuing education of all physicians to maintain professional skills. Maybe more importantly, he understands the need for a balanced approach to the problems that life brings to all of us.

We need these same sets of skills to help us approach the problems we may encounter as caregivers for the others in our lives, and as patients. How can we think "out of the box" to help get our aging parents to see the wisdom of moving to a living facility better suited to their needs in life? How do we sort through the various facts, political rhetoric and emotional issues to help medical groups, politicians and policymakers arrive at the best decisions for our country on ethical dilemmas such as abortion, stem cell research, genetic testing and other topics of the day?

Aristotle introduced the concept of the "joy of learning" over two thousand years ago in the age of great philosophers, artists and painters. Now, in our age of technology, we need teachers who will imbue in their students this enthusiasm for lifelong growth and learning. In 1987 Dr. Sherman Mellinkoff published a paper reviewing the teaching of the Art of Medicine in New Zealand, Australia and the United Kingdom. He found superb teachers of the Art of Medicine and cited a number of factors. The two of most importance were "Selection or recruitment of bright teachers who are anxious to remain students all their lives and who also derive joy from teaching and an atmosphere of discovery—an ever-expanding search for truth and correction of error. . . ."

Fortunately, those responsible for licensing physicians recognize this fact. The Federation of Medical State Licensing Boards is promoting the concept of lifelong continuing medical education with periodic assessments of medical knowledge as a key part of their mission. Hopefully, physicians will, in the future, have the ability to assess their medical knowledge in their own specialty area themselves without fear of punitive action. If weaknesses or gaps in knowledge are identified, physicians will then have the ability to find specific courses or materials to help them correct this. What could be better for both physician and patient?

When I first left residency and entered Emergency Medicine fulltime, I would have to call many physicians in private practice to come admit their patients after I had evaluated the patients in the ER. I was appalled at times at how many older physicians had not kept up with the latest in medicine, and how they were failing to use some of the latest drugs or technologies. I was arrogant enough to think that I'd never get behind the times like some of these doctors had. I was just too smart and too dedicated to ever let that happen to me. Now, after more than thirty years since beginning medical school, I have had the opportunity to eat a big piece of humble pie. To keep up with the changes in medical knowledge is nigh unto impossible, especially when the practice of medicine takes so much of your time, and personal issues like family take the rest. It takes real work and continuous commitment to maintain clinical skills and preserve competency.

Surprisingly, almost all state medical boards require continuing medical education but do *not* require any demonstration of **competency.** Many specialty medical boards like Family Practice and Emergency Medicine now require periodic retesting for members in order to maintain their specialty certification. There is much more to be done to help physicians maintain competency, but many excellent efforts meet heavy resistance from physician groups. It's too threatening to many of them now but with consumer and regulatory pressure, it one day will become reality. The key is assessment without punitive action, unless identified deficiencies are not corrected over a specified period of time.

We need to become involved and to take a stand. As healthcare professionals, we need to tell other physicians and our own professional organizations that we care about competency. Collectively, we need to learn from the mistakes of the past or we truly will be doomed to repeat them.

Commitment to Lifelong Learning—Questions

1. What can I do to maintain my skills in my own profession?
2. Are there performance assessment tools available to assess my level of competency?
3. What can I do to better educate myself and keep my mind working?
4. What things am I curious about in life and how do I harness that interest to stimulate my continued learning?
5. How do I help develop my ability to think "out of the box"?
6. What books or educational materials are available to help me solve the problems that confront me most frequently?
7. What people can serve as resources to help me or from whom I can learn?
8. How do I get involved in issues affecting medicine in my area or in my local hospital?

Our minds are the most valuable gift that God has given us. We have to keep them stimulated to use them most effectively. Cultivate your curiosity. Search out people and educational resources to help you grow constantly. A shark that doesn't keep swimming will die. A person who doesn't keep growing will die inside. Remember the old advertisement from the United Negro College Fund, "A mind is a terrible thing to waste." Don't let the beautiful, unique gift of your mind go to waste.

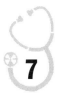

7

Women, Sex and the Internet

Dr. Maura Loftus was an irreverent, unconventional, motherly looking, middle-aged gynecologist who was this month's attending physician on the women's medical service. She was no-nonsense when it came to the women under her care, and expected both male and female residents and students to be extremely knowledgeable about women's issues. She was especially demanding of the female students because she felt that female patients expected more from doctors of the same gender.

She was addressing the entire staff on morning rounds on the first day of the month. The senior residents had just given the group a recap of all the women on the inpatient hospital service and soon most of the group were going to the ob-gyn clinic to see patients. "Welcome to the Women's Health Service. You'll be seeing a lot of me and I'll be asking you some very uncomfortable questions because I want you to be comfortable talking about those same issues with your patients. Most of the questions revolve around sex and the female anatomy. Thank God, some of you male students just woke up. I thought some of you were dead. This won't be like it was for you in college. I actually expect all of you to know the real truth about sex and the female anatomy, and not the stuff you learned from *Playboy*. Yeah, I know. You just bought them for the stories."

The entire group roared with laughter, except a couple of students who turned slightly pink with embarrassment. Dr. Loftus continued when the noise died down. "All of you are going to see a lot of pregnant women during these next two months. I expect every one of those women to be strongly encouraged to attend childbirth classes. If they aren't signed up for class yet, then they should be prompted to do so on every visit until they deliver. Does anyone have any idea why I want women to take these childbirth classes? Don't be bashful, men."

One of the fourth-year male residents bravely raised his hand. "What's your name, student?" Dr. Loftus asked.

"Frank Zinke, ma'am, and I have to say that I signed up for this rotation because I heard so many good things about your teaching."

Dr. Loftus smiled coyly and then asked softly, "Dr. Zinke, do you know the difference between a brown-noser and an ass-kisser?"

"Uh, no, ma'am. I don't."

"Well, it's depth perception. Now, stop trying to butter me up and answer my question."

The group erupted in laughter, because unknown to Dr. Loftus, Zinke had been known as a real suck-up in med school.

Zinke hurriedly answered. "The women will learn more about their pregnancy and delivery and they'll get a chance to meet and share information with other parents."

"Good; and why's that important?"

"You can learn some very practical tips to make your pregnancy and labor easier, especially if others have tried and experienced them."

"Anyone else have other reasons to take these classes? No? Well, what about the fathers? The classes help fathers and other family members become more involved in the pregnancy. Likewise, by having trained professionals teach these classes, many of the parents get answers to questions that they might not think of until it's too late. Finally, and most importantly, training in childbirth has been proven to improve a mother's chances for a less strenuous, shorter labor and to reduce the need for pain medicines. A big part of a physician's job is to educate and encourage patients to do the right things for their health, because you sure can't make them do it."

With that, the group broke up and headed for clinic. The Student felt a bit uncomfortable and very uncertain; he had never known anyone who'd been pregnant and, if the truth were known, he had very little experience dealing with women, either emotionally or sexually. Unfortunately, the women's clinic was packed on this particular day.

Dammit, could it get any worse? the Student thought. *I'm trapped here in the middle of an estrogen storm and I'm certainly not prepared for this. Thank God they paired me with me with Amy, one of my female classmates. At least, she's a bud. Plus, I've got a female resident as well so maybe I won't have to do too much today.*

The resident, an attractive young African-American woman, came over to the Student and his classmate and introduced herself. "Hi, I'm Dr. Peggy Strong. It's wall-to-wall people here today so let's get started. Here's how I'd like to work with you. I'd like for the two of you to go interview the patients first. Then, we'll go see them together after you've told me their stories. O.K.? Good. Student, you interview the first patient and then we'll let your colleague in crime do the next until we're done for the day. Come find me when you're ready to present." With that, the resident grabbed a chart and quickly entered a room.

The Student grabbed the next chart in line and with his classmate entered the patient's room. The patient was a woman in her early forties, and she was complaining of menstrual problems. He took the history in short order, found the resident, and quickly presented the woman's story. When he finished, the first question the resident asked was, "What's her sexual history and could she be pregnant?"

The Student was stunned and could barely utter a reply. "I didn't take a sexual history so I don't know whether or not she could be pregnant. I'm sorry. I just didn't think of pregnancy in a woman in her forties."

The resident shook her head incredulously. "Our sexuality is an integral part of each of us and deserves to be considered. <u>Always</u> take a sexual history as part of the workup of any problem involving the reproductive system in both men and women, and as part of any complete history and medical examination. Didn't they teach you any of this during basic medicine? When you don't specifically ask, you don't get the information."

Damn! The day did just get worse. She's right, of course, but it doesn't make me feel any less stupid.

The resident saw the woman and fortunately found that she could not have been pregnant because she hadn't had sex in a year. The patient's problems were directly related to the early changes of menopause. Once this was discussed with the patient, she decided to think about and research her options before beginning any hormone therapy at this visit. When they were alone again, his classmate, Amy, quickly asked the Student a question. "As a guy, what do you think are the reasons why women don't have sex?"

The Student immediately became visibly flustered. "Jeez, Amy, what kind of question is that? You know I'm no sexual expert on women."

"I know, I know. But as a woman, I think it's important that you understand some of the issues that we face when dealing with sexual issues. They may be some of the same reasons men avoid sex as well . . . as if any man would ever pass up the chance," she said with a smile on her face.

"Well, we're not all that way," the Student said grumpily.

"Oh yeah, I hate to tell you but my experience, and that of

my friends, is very much the other way. Look, for the most part, women approach sex very differently. For them it's a way of becoming more intimate with someone special. Men on the other hand will tell women what they want to hear just for the simple pleasure of the sexual act. Not that it's not fun, mind you," she said as she laughed again.

She continued. "I'm not putting you down but this past summer I did a special report on this for my Ph.D. project, and found that most male physicians are very uncomfortable asking women specific sexual questions, so in those rare cases where they do ask a question, they do it in very general terms like, 'Everything going all right at home?' Now, what kind of question is that? I'm giving you facts here. This is why many women prefer female physicians because they feel like they have a better chance of being listened to and of being understood. Again, back to my question. What are some of the reasons that keep women from enjoying or having sex?"

The Student thought for a minute before replying. "Some of the obvious reasons have to be fear of pregnancy or fear of disease. Another might be aging or the feeling of not being attractive. And finally, I'd have to guess is that they just don't like the person."

"Pretty good. Those are some of the reasons. I personally think you can divide the reasons into physiologic and emotional. As physicians, we need to deal with both, and the physical reasons are sometimes easier and quicker to identify but only if we ask the right questions. When a woman has hormonal changes, such as menopause or with her menstrual cycle, she may not lubricate as well or her vagina may be dry. This is why hormones in menopause help women feel so much better. There may be physical abnormalities that cause women pain with intercourse, or it may be a lack of stimulation during sex. Contrary to what many men may feel, a women's idea of foreplay starts long before the physical activity begins. It's how she's treated prior to getting into bed

Hey babe, after you get the kids to bed slip on that teddy I bought you because I'll be right up after the game is over.

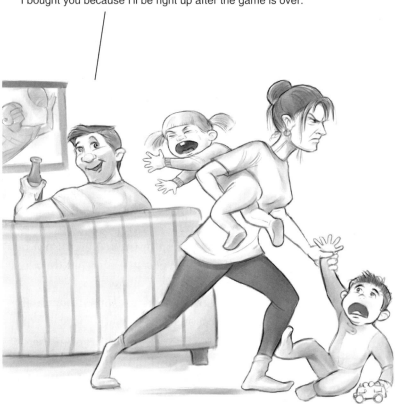

that makes all the difference in her enjoyment. 'Lie down, I think I love you,' does not constitute foreplay for women.

"Besides poor communication and general lack of intimacy, other emotional reasons that could affect a woman's response to sex might be related to bad experiences in the past, such as sexual abuse. There are just so many factors that could come into play. It's often a woman's gynecologist who discusses these issues with her. Over time, they build up a relationship characterized by a high level of trust and openness. That's why women have been heard to say, somewhat in jest, that they'd rather give up their husbands than their gynecologists." Amy stopped and looked at the Student. "Does this help any?"

The Student appeared somewhat dazed. "Yeah, it sure does. I just didn't realize that it was all that complicated. I just thought sex was sex. It does help me to understand why our resident crawled all over me before when I didn't ask some basic questions. I'm not sure I would have learned any of this if you hadn't been friend enough to share it with me. Thanks, Amy. It makes me wonder if some of the other guys in our class will ever learn any of this."

She smiled appreciatively and then got an impish grin on her face. She got close to the Student and whispered coyly, "Hey, do you think size matters in sex?"

The Student's face and neck instantly turned red. "Good God, Amy, what are you trying to do to me? How would I know if size makes a difference?"

In a most serious voice she said, "Just remember, you can't churn butter with a toothpick." She then laughed uproariously and ran off to see another patient.

Nothing terribly bad happened to the Student for the remainder of the clinic but he was still left with tremendous feelings of both discomfort and inadequacy. Learning about women was not going to be easy. He wasn't sure that time alone would make him feel any better. He smiled to himself as he thought about how his Dad was always making jokes about not understanding his Mom, even after being together for so long. As he was thinking about it all, he was paged to the ER. He was part of the team that was on call that day for the women's health service.

When he got to the ER, another of the female residents, Dr. Helen Chickering, greeted him. "Hi, I'm just going in to see a seventeen-year-old girl who came to the hospital complaining of abdominal pain. The ER doctor has done the initial workup and thinks she has PID, or pelvic inflammatory disease. Let's go talk to her."

Dr. Chickering had a reputation among the students for being one of the better housestaff teachers. She was a bit older than her other residents at the same level, since she had been a television reporter before coming to medical school. She was funny and irreverent but great with patients. She and the Student proceeded to interview the young girl. It turned out that she had had a number of sexual partners in high school. She had previously been treated for a trichomonas infection, but had never told her partner about it. She occasionally used condoms but not all the time, because she claimed the guys didn't like them. One of them had told her that it was like "showering in a raincoat." She knew about AIDS but thought it wouldn't happen to her. She had heard about sexually transmitted diseases, or STDs, but thought those didn't happen to "nice" girls.

The Student left the exam room in a somber mood. *How could she not use protection in this day and age, especially with all the information about HIV infection on TV and in the magazines and newspapers? Has she been living on some desert island? How could she be so stupid?*

Dr. Chickering was clearly angry. "I am so damned mad and so tired of seeing this same kind of stuff. When are these kids going to learn that it only takes a single sexual encounter to get a disease that can kill them, or that stays with them for the rest of their lives? What makes them think that they are immune or that it only happens to 'other' girls? It's so frustrating to treat them and then know that they're going to go back out and have sex again. At least, use a damned condom. Don't they learn anything about STDs?"

Chickering paged the attending that was on call for the weekend so that she could present the case to her, since it was likely to be an admission. Dr. Christine Dumas had a unique position on the women's health service. She only worked part time, two full weekends a month. She had two small children and wanted to spend more time with them at home while they were young. The women's health group had worked with a number of women over the years to make accommodations in their schedules because of personal family demands and had taken a great deal of heat from the rest of the medical school administration and faculty for it. It was a departmental decision; they wanted to create something different from other institutions because they didn't want to lose good people from the active practice of medicine.

The resident presented the case quickly to Dr. Dumas. "This seventeen-year-old girl has abdominal pain without pregnancy. She is sexually active. She is tender to touch both over the ovaries and when the uterus is moved. Smear of the vaginal fluid demonstrates trichomonas and there are herpetic appearing lesions on the external vagina. I believe she has PID, and because she's febrile, I'd like to admit her for IV antibiotics until she is less toxic."

Dr. Dumas reacted angrily as well. "Dammit! These kids have the bodies with all the equipment but they don't have the user's manual that tells them how to use it safely or properly. I hate to hear about these kinds of cases. Sure, let's admit her and let's see if we can spend some time trying to educate her how to reduce her risks. Did she suspect that she might be infected?"

"She admitted that it could be possible, as she'd been

treated in the past, but never followed up to make sure she was infection-free. The other fact that I omitted was that she doesn't require her partners to use condoms but I thought that was kind of obvious."

"O.K., let's get her going. If you have any problems give me a call. While you're writing the admission orders, I'll go talk to her and just listen to what else is going on here. Experience tells me that there's some other dynamic underlying her problem. It could be family, a drug issue or some esteem problem but today, I'm so concerned that these young girls imitate these rock stars like Britney Spears and Christina Aguilera. They want to grow up too fast and don't really enjoy these years that should be so carefree. Until we get to the bottom of this, the patient may continue some of her high-risk behaviors. Thanks for calling me."

When Dr. Dumas returned, she reported to the group that there were a number of other issues plaguing the young girl but she was steamed about another issue. "Sometimes I wish the Internet had never been invented. It's such a two-edged sword. It's great for disseminating information and is giving people access to untold amounts of knowledge like no other previous period in the history of mankind, but dammit, some of the information put out on websites and found in chat rooms is 100 percent bullshit."

Dr. Chickering looked at the attending almost in shock before replying, "What happened in there? I never hear you curse. You're like my mother. When I hear you use a four-letter word, it's serious."

"Oh, you're right. I don't like to use those kind of words but some of the medical misinformation that's found on the Internet is taken as truth by the unsuspecting, or those not able to evaluate this junk against more scientifically solid sites. You really have to be an informed consumer, and our young lady definitely was not." The attending paused to take a sip of her drink before continuing.

"Our patient has been logging onto a number of websites that cater to teens and young adults, but those more on the fringe. She got some information from some of the chat room 'experts' that douching after sex with vinegar would keep her from getting any STDs and lessen the chances of getting pregnant. She was on the pill so that didn't worry her. The other little bit of wonderful advice that she got was that condoms weren't all that effective in preventing disease, since some of the people in these chat rooms got infected even when using them on occasion. Of course they did. They didn't use them all the time and they probably didn't use them properly. No big surprise that they got infected. I wish they could monitor some of these sites for misinformation but I know it's a pipe dream and totally unrealistic. Hopefully, the good outweighs the bad. Enough of my ravings, let's get her admitted and I'll see you guys later. Call me if you need me."

As the team continued its workup of this patient, it got another page for a consult elsewhere in the hospital. It looked like it was going to be a long night.

✧ Perspectives for Doctors ✧

Failure to take a good sexual history in both men and women is one of the most common mistakes made by even experienced physicians. An AMA survey of physicians' history-taking practices revealed that only about 15% of doctors took even a cursory sexual history. In those doctors who took good histories, patients had sexual concerns over 50% of the time. This should come as no surprise. The sexual drive is one of the strongest that mankind, both men and women, possess; it's the one needed to keep the human race going. To keep the subject taboo or relegate sexual education to popular magazines such as *Cosmopolitan* and *Playboy* doesn't help anyone. Who better to talk about true sexual concerns than a doctor and his or her patient?

There are so many physiologic or biologic reasons for sexual problems that a doctor is usually the best person to address these issues. A patient often comes to the doctor with an underlying sexual issue but may not know how to raise the issue, or may often be afraid or embarrassed to discuss the issue. Frequently, the doctor has a great opportunity to discuss these issues since so many medicines can affect sexual functioning, but if the patient isn't asked about them, he or she could perhaps think problems are part of normal aging, or a side effect they just have to live with.

I will always remember a sixty-five-year-old man I saw in the ER for high blood pressure one night. His doctor already had him taking a couple of blood pressure medicines but he had stopped one of his medicines recently and his BP had shot back up. He always knew when his pressure was elevated because he developed headaches (most people have NO symptoms when their blood pressure goes up, and that's why it's known as the "silent killer"). After going through my workup, I spoke to him about the need to take his medicine regularly, because the blood pressure being high put him at increased risk for heart attack and stroke. I was so proud of myself for such a good lecture. He said he would and as I was leaving, I luckily asked him, "Why did you stop taking your medicine?"

He told me, "It doesn't sit well with me."

Fortunately, I asked him what that meant. "Well, it affects my manhood." Then I knew what his real problem was.

"You mean you can't get it up when you take this medicine."

"Yeah, doc. That's it exactly. You know, my wife and I still enjoy sex and I hate to miss out, so I stop my medicine sometimes."

I explained to him that this was a very well known side effect of the blood pressure medicine that he was taking, and that we could put him on something else that would control his pressure while avoiding these side effects. I learned a couple of things that evening. First, don't assume that a person's medicines have no side effects. Always ask patients about whether or not they are experiencing specific known side effects of that particular medicine. Don't wait for them to volunteer the information because they are often too embarrassed to do so. Second, "just because there's snow on the chimney, don't assume there's no heat in the fireplace." People are sexually active up into their eighties in many cases, so don't downplay the importance of sex as people age. These were two valuable lessons that served me extremely well over the years.

But is it totally the doctor's role to bring up all the issues of concern? Absolutely not. If patients are to have their needs met, they must learn to take responsibility for their own health. They need to speak up and share with their doctors the problems that are bothering them. Doctors and other healthcare professionals are not mind readers. They can only know of something because the patient shared the facts or issues with them.

Selectively sharing information with different healthcare providers is one of the things that I've seen happen in medicine, time and time again, and it's especially frustrating if it happens to you. As a student and resident, I experienced this, and I have spoken to many other doctors who went through the same thing. Here's how it would go: As a student, I'd go in and interview a patient and get one story. The resident would go in separately and get another story. Finally, when the attending would interview the patient in front of the entire group, the patient would often provide very different answers to the same questions that we had asked previously. It was extremely embarrassing and it made us appear that we had never asked the questions we actually did. The attending physicians would always know the true situation because it had happened to them when they were younger as well.

Why do patients hold back information or change their stories? Could they be confused by how questions are asked? Sometimes they gave a different answer to please the attending physician. Some patients tell the doctor what they think he or she wants to hear. Regardless, the best advice for patients is to be as truthful as possible on every occasion. Failure to do so can result in performing the wrong or unneeded testing, or worse, the wrong diagnosis.

Even though our society seems to sell sex constantly on TV, the movies, and in magazine and newspaper ads, talking about sex in an open and educational manner seems to be almost taboo. There is very little emphasis placed on sex education in the course of a medical education. So where do doctors get the sexual information they pass on to patients? Unless a physician is particularly interested in the subject, he or she gets very little from the formal medical educational system. Doctors are a very conservative group as a whole, and freely discussing sex is not easy for most. If a physician is uncomfortable with the subject and knows that he or she is not very knowledgeable about it, then he is not very likely to bring up the subject in the course of a medical examination.

Let's look at erectile dysfunction (ED) in men as a good example of physicians not identifying or dealing with a problem that surely existed before the manufacturers of Viagra made it acceptable to openly talk about it. Pfizer, the manufacturer of Viagra, spends millions of dollars annually, advertising directly to consumers and talking very forthrightly about the problem of ED. If ED is not a problem, then why is Viagra one of the largest selling drugs on the legitimate U.S. market, as well as on the black market? This problem existed for years but I rarely saw it mentioned in any continuing medical education seminars. The message for patients becomes clear. If it's an issue for you, you have to become proactive and raise the issue with your doctor yourself.

Finally, the number of cases of sexually transmitted diseases, or STDs, continues to increase despite costly educational efforts to reduce their numbers. There are over twenty-five STDs, with HIV, herpes and hepatitis getting the most attention, but the "old traditional" STDs, such as gonorrhea and syphilis, are present in ever-increasing numbers as well. The use of condoms can prevent the spread of these infections but many men refuse to use them for many obscure reasons, none of which make any sense. Women need to be taught to take control in these situations. In the Greek play, *Lysistrata*, women refused to have sex until all war was stopped. Well, the battle with STDs is raging and we're not winning with the present strategy. We need to educate our young people to abstain but when they don't, to use a condom. *You want me. You use a condom. No sex without latex.*

During one of my most recent shifts in the ER, I saw a fourteen-year-old girl with HIV in one room, and my next patient was a fifteen-year-old boy also with HIV infection. The nurses told me that the young girl had gotten infected from the boy, who was her boyfriend. He had gotten HIV from an infected needle. They were both bright kids from good families. What a preventable tragedy! That night I went home and hugged my then-teenaged girls.

A recent book written by a woman physician carefully documents that not a single case of HIV has occurred in the legal brothels in Nevada over the last twelve years because of the required use of condoms by the prostitutes working there. This is a true public health success and shows the power of prevention when done properly. It's up to all of us to look out for ourselves.

Here's a statistic that I found astonishing. By the year 2015, 50% of women in the U.S. will be menopausal. Huge numbers of Baby Boomer women will be aging. The future of medicine has changed drastically over the past decade because the composition of medical school classes has changed dramatically in the same time period. In many medical schools, women now compose 50% or more of the class makeup. This means that more and more residency slots will be going to women who might not be willing to work in the same way men have done in the past. A good example of this is the fact that only 30% of women physicians completing a general surgical residency are still in practice while 90% of men are in practice.

Traditional medicine has not really embraced those who want to practice medicine on a part-time basis. It's extremely unfortunate because many talented women (and men) have been lost to clinical practice. Many find administrative jobs or non-clinical jobs but this often leaves these physicians feeling less fulfilled. Medicine must find a way to accommodate these physicians. Patients must take an active role in noting their displeasure when a physician leaves a group because a part-time schedule can't be worked out for that physician.

The Internet has been a wonderful source of knowledge for all of us, and has opened wide the doors of information. Scientists use it to share information from all over the world. By unlocking the power of the Internet, patients can become as knowledgeable as their doctors on some subjects. No longer is the physician the sole source of medical knowledge. And for that reason, the dynamics of the doctor-patient relationship have changed forever. Let me issue one word of warning that's similar to the old Roman adage of "Caveat emptor" or "Let the buyer beware." Today, I believe the better saying where the Internet is concerned should be "Let the user beware." Just because it's in print doesn't make it the truth. Just look at what you read in the paper or what advertising would have you believe. We have to be extremely careful about what kind of information we get, and where and from whom we get it. Many people have biases or agendas when they write, report or issue studies. You might think that the American Tobacco Institute is an independent group promoting excellent research on smoking but instead it's a trade organization for big tobacco. Studies coming from there have to be viewed with an extremely jaundiced eye. We should always look at both sides of an issue to gain the proper perspective. There are two sides to a story and the truth probably lies somewhere in the middle. As the story above illustrates all too well, there is a great deal of misinformation or false information on the Internet, along with the vast majority of excellent, scientifically solid information. Here are some simple suggestions for evaluating medical information on the Internet:

Tips for Getting Medical Information from the Internet

1. Obtain your medical information from respected, universally accepted websites such as the Library of Congress, American Cancer Society, national medical specialty organizations, or similar groups.

2. Look to special-interest medical problem groups for legitimate information, e.g., those with Parkinson's disease can help others with the same problem and provide very specialized knowledge from people who have experienced the disease and its associated problems.

3. Validate whatever information you obtain from peripheral sites at another source, just to be as safe as possible. Reporters verify their sources and so should you.

4. Ask others researching a similar medical problem which websites have been most helpful for them.

5. Explore alternative medicine sources for helpful information. Traditional medicine certainly doesn't have all the answers.
6. If something looks too good to be true or too simple, it probably is.
7. Use your brain. Review the scientific evidence. Does it make sense?

8

Laughter is the Best Medicine—Humor and Healing

Q. —What do they call the person who graduates last in their medical school class?

A. —Doctor

"The Art of Medicine consists of amusing the patient while nature cures the disease."

–Voltaire

The Advisor had asked the Student to meet him at 6:30 p.m. in front of the hospital and to wear a coat and tie. He was very mysterious about the whole thing and refused to tell him anything more than what to wear. While waiting, the Student began to think about all that he'd experienced in the months since starting his visits with the Advisor. The old guy was beginning to grow on him, and he couldn't exactly figure out why. Now, he actually found himself looking forward to their meetings, since he never knew what he'd be experiencing next. His thoughts were suddenly interrupted by a car horn. "Oogha, Oogha." Somehow, he knew it could only be one person driving a car making that unusual sound. What surprised him, however, was the sight of the beautiful old Porsche that his Advisor was driving.

What a car! I've never seen anything like it, the Student thought. *The old guy might be a ham sandwich short of a picnic in the reality department but he certainly was full of surprises.*

The Student got into the car while his eyes inspected every inch of the restored interior.

"This is absolutely beautiful!" he gushed admiringly. "It must have cost a fortune."

"Nope, did it all myself in my spare time," responded the Advisor proudly. "I was out one day jogging and spotted this up on blocks in someone's yard. I stopped, knocked on the door, and told the owner that I wanted to buy his rusted, wrecked, shell of a car for a $1000. We eventually settled on $1500. It took me almost three years of part-time work to restore it but you can see the end result. It was truly a labor of love for me. Working with my hands is fun for me, and it kept me around the house so that I was closer to my family. One day, hopefully, you'll experience for yourself that family is the greatest support you can have, but it takes being there to make it work. Unfortunately, being a surgeon requires a great deal of time away from them so you have to look for ways to get your recreation and still be around.

"Curious about where we're going tonight, Student?" the Advisor inquired.

"Yeah, I have to admit, I thought about it all day. You were so mysterious. I couldn't figure out why the plans for tonight were such a secret. It really did get my curiosity going. OK, time for you to come clean."

"Fair enough," replied the Advisor with a huge smile.

"We're going to the County Medical Society meeting to hear a very special visiting physician speak. How's that sound?"

"You really want me to be honest?" the Student inquired.

"Sure, I always do. What kind of a relationship would we have if you couldn't be honest with me?"

The Student thought for a minute and then replied somewhat irritably. "Frankly, it doesn't sound all that appealing to me. I've been working pretty hard on my medical rotation. Until you called, my plans for the evening called for me to be sitting down at the Graduate pub with some friends and putting down some tall ones while watching the Duke-Carolina basketball game on TV."

"Fair enough," countered the Advisor. "I promise you the evening won't be as dull as you're imagining it right now."

They rode in silence for a few minutes before the Advisor spoke. "Do you know when humor began to play an important part in a society's culture?" he asked.

Where is this guy coming from? Who cares? I don't want to be here going to some stupid, stodgy lecture designed to put me to sleep. I want to watch Coach K and the Dukies kicking some serious Tar Heel butt. Buy a vowel and get a clue, please. I am NOT interested in more of your ancient history lessons. The Student smiled slightly while thinking. *Bet the old guy will be surprised when I know the answer to this one.*

"I know that you think you got me on that one but I happened to be watching the movie *Shakespeare in Love* the other night so I know that it was the Middle Ages when humor became important to a society. They even had court jesters to keep people laughing. Not bad, huh?"

"Not bad, but not good either," chided the Advisor. "Actually, we have records going back to the time of the Ancient Egyptians, as well as the Greeks in Hippocrates's time, that support the idea that humor in these societies was seen as an important ingredient in a person's health. It's actually been an essential part of every culture and every society until the present. Certain Indian tribes had medicine men whose job was to safeguard the humor of the society. Don't forget Norman Cousin's book titled *Anatomy of an Illness,* in which he described the positive effects that humor had on his efforts to deal with his ankylosing spondylitis. From the most primitive cultures to the present, humor is clearly one of the keys to our survival."

The Advisor paused to let his Student process his comments and then continued. "Let me give you a practical example to illustrate my point. When researchers interviewed people who've survived terrible situations like concentration camps, disasters, cancer, and wars, they found certain common factors in almost all of them—a belief in a Higher Power, a sense of altruism, a support system of family or friends, and the ability to find humor in the everyday despite the horror around them. Humor helps us get through some high-stress situations. It's one of the reasons you find such dark humor in ERs and in operating rooms. And think about it: if we need it, then our patients may need it even more because they have to endure some pretty terrible things. They don't need doctors who don't have a sense of humor or can't laugh at themselves."

About then they pulled up to the front of the hotel where the County Medical Society meeting was being held. Before exiting the car, the Advisor pulled some papers from his pocket and handed them to the Student.

"I brought you an article to read. Why don't you look at it while I park the car? Dr. Robert Rakel is one of this country's leading educators in the field of Family Practice. He's authored four major textbooks and has written a number of excellent articles about a physician's need for compassion, understanding and a sense of humor when dealing with patients. I'd like for you to take a minute and read it now because it will help to put this evening's program into perspective for you."

The Advisor's beeper went off about that time. He looked down at his pager and then said, "Sorry, but I've got to return this page right away. I'm on call tonight for general surgery. We can discuss the article further over dinner."

About twenty minutes later, the Advisor returned and asked the Student, "Have you ever heard of Dr. Steve Allen?"

"Is this a trick question? Because even I know that Steve Allen was some old comedian who died recently," the Student answered.

"Student, one nice thing about youth: You may be wrong but you're never in doubt. Dr. Steve Allen, Jr., is a highly respected Family Physician on the faculty at SUNY-Upstate, who also happens to be a comedian, magician and juggler. He's decided that one of his teaching roles is to educate his fellow physicians on the need to laugh for both themselves and their patients' benefit. It's one of the reasons I had you read Dr. Rakel's article. He and Dr. Allen are doctors who understand the need for physicians to get down off their pedestals to laugh and share their humanity with their fellow man.

"Dr. Allen is the principal speaker—or in his case—entertainer after dinner this evening. I thought you might enjoy a different look at medicine, not to mention meeting some of the other doctors in our town. It's a different world outside the ivory tower of the medical school, and it's important that you understand and experience it. This is one of the reasons I encourage all my students to take externships away from the medical center and out in the community somewhere."

At that moment, they arrived at the meeting room where the evening's events were being held. The Advisor motioned the Student to a table with two empty chairs. An attractive woman in her mid-thirties turned as they approached and laughingly said, " Watch out for your wallets everyone, the Old Guy is here."

The Advisor just chuckled and said, "Dr. Meg Humphrey was one of my Advisees in the past, and somehow or another, made it out of residency and into the best ENT practice in town. She's a wonderful example of the old saying that 'Miracles do happen every day.' She's also one of the funniest and most irreverent women I've ever met."

Dr. Humphrey just laughed before quickly introducing the rest of the table to the Student. The remainder of the group consisted of a general surgeon, an orthopedist and a pediatrician. The dinner came almost immediately and the conversation took the course of a general update on news of families and friends while everyone ate. It didn't take long before the conversation turned to the subject of the evening, and Dr. Humphrey took the lead. "Since we're here to laugh tonight and put things into perspective, here's one that a patient told me today.

"A woman accompanied her husband to the doctor's office. After the checkup, the doctor took the wife aside and told her, 'If you don't do the following, your husband will surely die:

1. Each morning, fix him a healthy breakfast and send him off to work in a good mood.
2. For dinner, fix an especially good meal and don't burden him with household chores.
3. Satisfy his every whim, like allowing him to play golf twice on the weekends.
4. Have sex with him several times a week.'

On the way home, the husband asked the wife what the doctor had said to her. She replied, 'You're going to die.'"

Everyone at the table roared, including the Student. The pediatrician, Dr. Steve West, told the group that he had been reading a book about humor and it contained a quote by Harriet Beecher Stowe that had caught his attention. "*A person without humor is like a wagon without springs, they are jolted by every bump in the road.*" The whole table nodded their heads in unison when he finished the quote.

The general surgeon, Dr. Tim Flynn, a funny Irishman

from Louisiana with a thick Cajun accent, spoke up next, "You know, I really believe that's true. I find in my own practice that those patients who have a sense of humor, and who can laugh about life and their particular situation, always do better than patients who lack that ability to find humor in life. In fact, I find my whole office practice runs better if we can all stop and laugh once in a while. I've even instituted a 'Laugh and Learn Lunch' session for all my staff once a month. It's a time when we all relax and laugh together while learning something fun that has nothing to do with medicine. No one would dare miss these. We all need to remember that our patients can sense our moods. If we're uptight, then it's tougher for them to open up to us. I want my patients to feel comfortable and at ease. I know there will be times when they are going to have to wait for a time despite my best efforts so they'll be in a lot better mood when I see them if they can laugh with my staff. I even have old comedy tapes playing in my waiting room."

Dr. West then mentioned how he had been a resident with the real Patch Adams and how he used laughter to defuse so many difficult situations. "He told me that it's all in how you approach things. If you look for humor, you'll find it, but you have to be open to it. Just look at Jay Leno's show. He finds humor in wedding announcements, personal ads and so many common things that we all miss . . . just because he's looking for it."

The Advisor entered the conversation at that point. "When one looks at many of the great leaders such as Lincoln, Churchill and others, they all had great senses of humor. They knew that they needed it to bear up under the tremendous pressures they faced in their jobs. I hate to admit it but it's one of the reasons I like all of you so much. You all know how to keep life and medicine in proper perspective. And to help you do that, here's a joke my brother, the orthopedist, just e-mailed me."

Q—"When is it safe to transfer a multiple trauma patient to the orthopedic service?"

A—"When the patient could survive for two weeks locked in a garage with only two gallons of water."

The whole table laughed again in appreciation of a joke that had a fair amount to truth to it. About that time, the president of the medical society got the group's attention and began the introductions of Dr. Allen. The program quickly got into full swing with the entire audience joining in with comments and heartfelt laughter.

Dr. Allen explained to the group how humor was essential to our survival and was indigenous to all cultures and races. Because this was a physicians' group, he provided some scientific studies to support the theory that humor stimulated the immune system and increased the level of endorphins in our brains. Endorphins were the morphine-like hormones that helped to decrease our stress and keep us mellow. He then went into some depth about the different types of humor and told a number of jokes to illustrate his points. Finally, he made the entire group get up and go through what he called Humorobics, an exercise to get people laughing by making funny faces and doing silly things.

After the program ended, the Advisor and Student said their goodbyes and made their way to the car. As they got closer to the car, the Advisor asked, "Would you like to drive home?"

"Would I? You'd better believe it, but what if something happens?"

"Don't worry; that's why I have insurance," the Advisor replied.

They both got in and the Student edged the car out of the parking space extra carefully. He then exited the garage and quickly moved onto the main downtown street.

"Well, was the evening what you expected, Student?"

The Student thought for a moment and then chuckled.

"Honestly, it was nothing like I expected but in a very good way. I couldn't get over how down to earth all the other doctors were, and Dr. Allen's presentation really rocked. It was the bomb. I can't remember when I laughed so much. It certainly gave me a different perspective on medicine. I'll have to admit that I didn't once think about the basketball game. Thanks for bringing me."

The Advisor smiled, reclined his seat and then spoke with great feeling, " No, thanks to you, Student. You just made this evening very special for me also."

With that, they drove home together in contented silence.

❖ *Perspectives for Doctors* ❖

When I was young boy, I used to pick up my mother's monthly copy of the *Reader's Digest*. I always looked forward to the great stories in there but one of the sections that I always read, without fail, was *Laughter, the Best Medicine.* That section contained some very funny jokes that you could actually repeat in mixed company. I always felt better after reading that section, and I never really understood why. Now, I think I do.

It's clear from medical research that humor has some very important and well-documented, beneficial, health effects. It lowers blood pressure, stimulates the immune system, decreases anxiety and raises levels of endorphins in our brain that help us to feel better. The connection between humor and health has been known for thousands of years and in a variety of cultures across the globe. The ancient Greeks and Romans all had funny men as a part of their efforts to help people feel better. The American Indians had a medicine man as well as a tribe clown. The English had their court jesters. Today, we go to comedy clubs to laugh at both the world around us and ourselves. It's all about helping us to forget our troubles and feel better. Dr. Thomas Sydenham, the great seventeenth century physician, may have expressed it best: *"The arrival of a good clown exercises more beneficial influence upon the health of a town than of twenty asses laden with drugs."*

Dr. Patch Adams, the real-life hero of the movie by the same name, is a doctor who is a social revolutionary and who has founded a free hospital known as the Gesundheit Institute in West Virginia. He believes strongly that humor is vital in healing the problems of individuals, communities and societies. He has tried throughout his career to bring humor to the hospital setting. Unfortunately, his efforts have often been derided because most administrators and staff seem to believe that a somber atmosphere is essential to healing when just the opposite is needed. The real effort should be focused on enhancing the positive in people's lives while learning to talk about the relationships that mean the most to people.

Corporate America could also use a healthy dose of humor in the workplace. It's clear from several good research papers that an office that can laugh and knows how to have fun at appropriate times is also more productive and less stressed. With most corporations cutting their work forces back, they are asking the remaining employees to do more with less help. Humor can do much to diffuse the stress that the added burdens bring. Plus, if you can't escape the job or the situation, humor helps to get you through a bad situation. Isn't that exactly the reason behind the humor found in operating rooms and ERs?

What's it take to get more humor in our lives? It takes perspective. The Roman, Epictetus, said, *"Man is not disturbed by events but by the view he takes of them."* Two people can go through the exact experience or event but the attitude, training and past experience of one versus the other can markedly change our perspective—and the resulting emotions that accompany it. Medical school can be viewed as a stressful, four-year, torture-filled drag, or it can be viewed as a wonderful,

How fish see fishing lures.

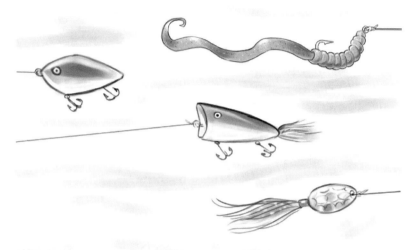

Such pretty colors! I could sit here and watch for hours.

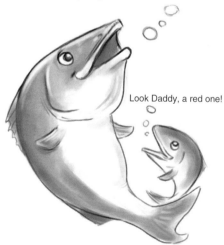

Look Daddy, a red one!

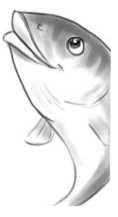

new learning experience that will change your life and bring you into contact with some special people. Which person do you think will do better throughout his or her four years of school? The same is true of any life experience. Think about how your perspective can change things, and work on improving the way you view life events. I've heard so many people say that the events of September 11, 2001, have helped provide perspective on what's really important in life. The focus should be on people and not things. Is the glass half-empty or half-full? How you feel is your choice.

Finally, I 'm going to ask you to do two things and keep them in mind as you go through life. First, What's on your JOY LIST? **Your Joy List is a list of things that have nourished and sustained you and given you a sense of joy in being alive.** Why is a Joy List so important? Because when times are tough, when you're feeling down, or when you're feeling sorry for yourself, think of your Joy List and things will definitely improve. Trust me, it works. I've shared this concept with many people during my talks on *Humor and Healing* and it's an immediate pick-me-upper for everyone present. Try it. What have you got to lose?

The second thing I 'm going to ask you to do is perform an exercise to help get rid of the Blues. Despite our best efforts, we all get down at times and we need something like our Joy List to get us out of our blue moods. I've asked people in my lectures to make a list of things they do to get rid of the Blues. I've compiled a Top 10 list of things that work for most people. The bottom line for you: Think what works for you and use it. Remember, *"Angels can fly because they take themselves so lightly."* We all need to do the same.

Top 10—How to Get Rid of the Blues

1. Call a loved one.
2. Look at your Joy List.

3. Exercise.
4. Watch a comedy tape or funny movie.
5. Read a good book.
6. Spend time with children.
7. Spend time with people who are happy.
8. Smile at people you don't know.
9. Do something crazy.
10. Visit someone in the hospital and realize your blessings.

Again, what have you got to lose? How you feel is your choice. Remember, the Art of Medicine is all about healing the mind, the body, and the spirit. A sense of humor and keeping things in perspective are integral to this end.

9

The General Medical Service

"A Generalist is a doctor who keeps knowing less and less about more and more until he knows nothing about everything.

"A Specialist on the other hand keeps knowing more and more about less and less until he knows everything about nothing."

–Anonymous

"Death is not a failure of medical science but the last act of life."

–Patch Adams, MD

It was Tuesday morning and that meant only one thing on the General Medical service—Grand Rounds. Twice a month the medical service had an in-depth presentation on some medical disease by either a visiting lecturer or an in-house faculty member. On one of the other Tuesdays, an interesting medical case involving a patient on the medical service was presented to all the faculty, residents and students. On the final Tuesday of the month, a morbidity and mortality (M&M) conference was held in which a death or poor outcome was reviewed with the entire medical staff.

Grand Rounds were considered very important occasions and a good deal of time was spent preparing the presentations for each week. Generally, the discussions were friendly and amiable, but on occasion, they became quite heated, especially when there were various options available for treating a particular disease. Sometimes the presenter could be embarrassed because of the way a case was handled or for failing to know the answers to some of the questions that were asked by the audience. So for presenters, the whole process could be extremely unnerving at times.

Dr. Bill Porter was the medical attending for the month and had instructed all the medical students on the importance of attending all the Grand Rounds presentations. "The primary purpose behind Grand Rounds is to educate everyone by learning from a variety of teachers, cases and in some instances, mistakes. Learning should be a lifelong experience for physicians, and Rounds is a great way to model learning from each other. No matter what your specialty, there is always something to learn because medicine is constantly changing."

Today's lecture was to be given by Dr. Patrick Ober, a Professor of Endocrinology at Wake Forest School of Medicine. Dr. Ober had won many teaching awards during his years in academia and believed that learning best occurred when the atmosphere was relaxed and there was a free exchange of ideas.

The Student was seated in the audience, as it was his second week on his medical rotation. He, along with all the other students on the medical service, was to go on rounds with Dr. Ober as part of the medical team later in the day.

I just hope to God that I don't get asked any questions today. That's all I need. I doubt I'll know the answer and I'll be embarrassed in front of the entire medical service. My name will be forever emblazoned on their memories so that they'll pick on me whenever they need a laugh.

Dr. Ober began his lecture on endocrinology with the pituitary gland and proceeded to work his way down the body until he reached the adrenal glands. It was a different approach to a well-known body system and kept the audience entranced for over an hour.

He finished his talk with one final point. "The zona glomerulosa is the outer layer of the adrenal cortex, and produces a hormone that regulates sodium and potassium, the body's important salts. The next layer is the zona fasciculata, which produces a hormone that regulates the level of glucose, the sugar that is the body's essential energy source. The inner layer is the zona reticularis, which produces hormones that are referred to as androgens, or sex hormones. I know this is a huge amount of information to carry around in your head, and it might seem overwhelming. In medicine, you'll find that you won't be able to use information effectively and accurately unless you have it organized in a manner that's accessible to you. Here's a clue that will help you to remember the three major functions of the adrenal gland as you go from the outer layer to the inner layer. The adrenals regulate salt, sugar and sex but how can you remember the order of these with little effort? Here's what I use. From out to in, remember salt, sugar and sex. The deeper you go, the sweeter it gets."

With that the audience roared and began to applaud. This would be a lecture that would be hard to top in the upcoming weeks. At the conclusion of the lecture, the medical team moved to the front of the auditorium to wait for Dr. Ober. They were heading to the medical floor to make rounds on the patients in the hospital for the next couple of hours. It was a chance to learn medicine from someone new that wasn't inhibited or constrained by any of the local politics often associated with medical care within a large medical center.

There were a total of fifteen medical team members in all, which included attending physicians, residents, medical students and nurses. They all entered the room of the first patient and quickly surrounded the bed of a somewhat obese middle-aged woman. The chief resident then began to speak, "Mrs. Lopez is a fifty-six-year-old divorced woman who presented in diabetic ketoacidosis three days ago. She's had Type II diabetes for years but had recently become refractory to oral medicines and diet. She was started on insulin therapy four months ago with better control of her diabetes. About ten days before her admission, she cut her foot while walking barefoot in her yard. The wound became infected. At the same time, she stopped taking her insulin because she'd run out and didn't get her prescription refilled. She was admitted with a blood sugar of 510 and with overt symptoms of confusion. We have since gotten her diabetes under control, and she is due to be discharged today, but only if she can demonstrate a good understanding of her condition and how to care for herself. Any questions?"

There was a moment of silence before one of the other residents asked a simple question that was easily answered. Mrs. Lopez just sat and smiled the entire time. Since the case seemed fairly straightforward, there were no more questions so the whole team filed out into the corridor and started to move to the next patient's room. At that point, Dr. Ober spoke up for the first time, "What were some of your observations about Mrs. Lopez while we were in her room?"

One of the other residents spoke up and said, "She seemed to be well hydrated and she had good oral intake according to the I and O chart. She was urinating frequently but that's not surprising in a diabetic."

The senior attending then said, "The infection on her foot looked like it was doing better because the skin on her foot was pink and healthy appearing."

Dr. Ober looked around the group but no one else offered any further comments. He paused before proceeding, "Did anyone notice what was **not** in Mrs. Lopez's room or at her bedside? There were no cards, no flowers and no personal items. Most people have one of those things in their rooms even on their first day in the hospital. What do you think that tells us about her family or her social support system? Does anyone have any idea about those?"

There was a moment of embarrassed silence before the second year resident spoke, "I think Mrs. Lopez is recently divorced, but I really didn't take a good family history. Sorry, I definitely overlooked it because things have been so busy lately."

"Thanks for your honesty. It's a good example for us all. Why don't we all go back into the room and ask some more questions?"

The entire entourage moved back into Mrs. Lopez's room and Dr. Ober took the lead. "Mrs. Lopez, is it OK if we ask you some more questions?"

"*Sí* . . . uh, I mean, yes."

With that, Dr. Ober began to dig into Mrs. Lopez's personal life. Her English was not the greatest but Dr. Ober used his little knowledge of Spanish to make it easier for her. It took some time but in the process he discovered many things that had significant bearing on this case. Her husband of many years was a long-standing alcoholic. Just recently, she had asked him to leave home because he was physically abusing their three children when he was drunk. Because of his departure, money was tighter than ever, so she tried to do without her medicine to save whatever dollars she could. She knew her foot was bad but she was hoping that her home remedies could get in under control. She didn't realize that diabetics could so easily get out of control when they had infections elsewhere in their body. She admitted that she was scared and didn't know how she would pay for her medicines once she got out of the hospital, much less pay for her hospital bill.

Once the questioning was completed, there was stunned silence as everyone filed from the room. A significant lesson had been learned that not many would forget. All were humbled by what they had failed to see and amazed by what a good clinician could learn by taking a complete, careful history.

Several more patients were seen before Dr. Ober left to meet with the dean and his staff for lunch. At that point, Dr. Porter took over to see the final few patients with the group. The last patient of the morning was a young woman transferred from the OB-GYN service in the middle of the night. The resident on call the night before who had admitted the patient made the presentation to the group.

"Mrs. Woodward is a forty-five-year-old, married white female who was transferred to the medical service from the gynecology group last night. She has had a total hysterectomy secondary to ovarian cancer about two years ago. She has undergone radiation and is now on her second course of chemotherapy. She was admitted to the medical service because of persistent, uncontrollable vomiting secondary to the chemotherapy, and for her anemia and electrolyte imbalances. I was told by the oncology group that they have little left to offer Mrs. Woodward so once we get her vomiting under control, we can only offer palliative care." At that, the obviously tired resident looked around the group to see if there were any questions.

Dr. Porter also looked around the group before asking, "What has Mrs. Woodward been told by the oncologists? Does she know that this is the beginning of the end?"

The resident sighed wearily before replying, "To be honest, I was so busy that I didn't go into it with her, and I forgot to ask the resident on OB-GYN when she was being transferred. I'll check into that and put a note on the chart."

Dr. Porter then addressed the entire group. "There are many issues to face when a patient is dying, and some of the biggest revolve around communication with the patient and his or her family. Patients need time to come to terms with their own death. If any of you have not read Dr. Elizabeth Kubler-Ross's book, *On Death and Dying*, it's an excellent resource that every physician should read before caring for terminally ill patients. It will help you to understand the various emotional stages that most patients go through as they face a potentially life ending disease. There's also an excellent play, and now a movie, titled *Wit* that deals with the medical indignities heaped on a dying cancer patient at the end of her life. The play provides amazing insights into a terminal patient's end of life issues. I strongly recommend getting the video and watching it."

Dr. Porter wasn't sure if they really understood what he was talking about or not, but he continued anyway. "Patients who are dying need to feel cared for, but also want to feel in control. There are a number of end-of-life issues that they, and their loved ones, need to deal with, such as when, or if, to get hospice involved. Should the patient be resuscitated if his heart should stop, or if she stops breathing? What about pain control? Does he want to die at home, or in the hospital? It may surprise you but most patient surveys indicate that about 80% of patients would prefer to die at home rather than in the hospital. Yet, despite their wishes, the actual reality of the situation is that they usually end up dying in the hospital. How can we, as physicians, help with this disconnect? This is one of the great benefits of the hospice movement. It helps families care for their loved ones at home in a personal, meaningful way so that death becomes a natural part of life, just like birth. I won't kid you. These are not easy issues to talk about, and because of that, many doctors and healthcare professionals shy away from them. I personally believe that failing to talk about them with patients and their families is akin to malpractice."

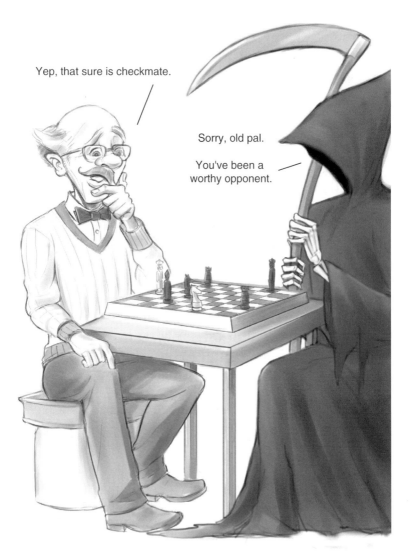

Dr. Porter again paused and studied the group. That last statement had really gotten their attention. "Just think about how you'd like to see one of your loved ones treated, or even better, how you'd like to be treated. Patients need to be given the choices available for their care and then, they need to be given the autonomy to make the decisions that are right for them. Only then will they become participants in their own care. It might not be what you and I would choose, but it's right for them. You keep this in mind, and you'll never go wrong. Now, let's go in and see Mrs. Woodward."

The group had now dwindled to about nine members, but it was still sizable as they entered the small hospital room. Mrs. Woodward was propped up in bed with a couple of pillows and looked quite pale, and obviously wasted. All could see that the cancer was winning the battle with the patient. Dr. Porter immediately sat down on the bed, held her hand, and introduced himself and the group. "Looks like you're a little tired today?"

She smiled wearily before replying, "Some of your friends here kept me up a great deal of the night talking and drawing blood. Don't you think you could do with a little less blood? I've got a bad feeling that I'm going to need all that I've got."

Dr. Porter smiled also. "Maybe we could. I'll see what we can do but we do have to see how you're doing, don't we?"

Mrs. Woodward picked her head up and looked Dr. Porter directly in the eye. "Don't kid me, doctor. We both know that I'm dying, and that none of you have much to offer me. I feel like a pincushion, I've been stuck so much lately. I'm worn out and don't have any fight left, so what is all this really going to do for me? Isn't it a bit academic?"

The tension in the room was almost palpable and everyone in the group was glad that it wasn't them sitting on the bed being confronted by the patient. None of them had seen this kind of interaction between doctor and patient before while on the medical service.

Dr. Porter didn't bat an eye as he replied, "Yes, you are dying, and I don't have any miracle cures in my bag of tricks. I agree with you that I see no need to continue some of the chemotherapy that you've been undergoing. We do need to take some blood occasionally so that we can try to make you more comfortable, but that's also something we can talk about at a later time. What I can do for you is a number of things. I can give you some options about your care and treatment. I can make you more comfortable so that you don't feel any pain, and I can spend time with you to listen, and help you on this last part of your life's journey. I'll personally make that commitment to you."

Mrs. Woodward continued to look Dr. Porter in the eye for another minute while not one of the other nine persons in the room moved or uttered a sound. She then allowed her face to break into a small smile. "You're a good man, Dr. Porter. I didn't want any bullshit, and you didn't give me any. I'm glad you're my doctor."

Dr. Porter laughed, stood up, and before he left the room said, "I'm glad I'm your doctor too, Mrs. Woodward. See you tomorrow."

The group filed out silently. All knew they had glimpsed a rare encounter and learned a lesson in the Art of Medicine that would stick with them for a lifetime.

Dr. Porter stopped the group further down the hall. "You all have just met a brave woman who will need our visits each day. You'd all profit by spending some time with her and just listening. Ask her about her life and listen to her story. She needs time to tell it. It's easy to avoid someone who's dying because it makes us all uncomfortable as it could be viewed as our failure. It's hard for us all to remember that it's as normal a part of life as being born is." Dr. Porter then dismissed the residents so that they could finish writing orders before medical clinic began that afternoon. Dr. Porter then reminded the medical students "Don't forget that all the medical students on the Orange and Blue rotations are rounding with Dr. Ober this afternoon. Meet him in front of the ICU at one o'clock."

Later that afternoon eight medical students and eight residents met in front of the ICU. Dr. Ober was on time and was joined by this month's attending on the ICU, Dr. Byron Williams. Dr. Williams was a great athlete in his college days and still stayed in shape by competing with his five sons in various sports. He was a cardiologist who loved teaching and had won numerous teaching awards over the years. They all entered the ICU and immediately went to the bed of the first patient.

Neither the Student nor his classmates had ever been inside the ICU before. The first thing that hit them all was the powerful odors of antiseptic, blood and body fluids. They weren't necessarily offensive, but were pervasive, and a bit unsettling. Their senses of hearing were the next to be assailed. There was the constant beeping and pinging of various kinds of monitors, plus the hissing of the bellows on what appeared to be a mandatory respirator attached to every patient in the unit. There were people everywhere . . . all providing some service to the different patients. The Student would later learn that these were nurses, respiratory therapists, physical therapists, as well as physicians of all sorts, who were there to consult on the patients. All of this was overwhelming.

How do the patients stand it? I could never sleep with all the noise, the bright lights and the people. Get me out of here and back to radiology. This is insanity. I bet they're all dying to get out of here. Ooh, sick joke! Not very funny.

The voice of the second-year medical resident beginning the usual recitation on a patient snapped the Student back to the present. "Mr. Payne is a fifty-five-year-old white male who recently had surgery for a number of internal injuries suffered in an auto accident. He was talking on his cell phone when he ran into the rear of another car that had stopped at a light. He had also stupidly forgotten to wear his seat belt. He had a ruptured spleen and lacerated liver as well as a compound fracture of his right leg. He came through surgery successfully but we couldn't get him off the respirator thanks to his forty-year history of smoking. He developed DT's—uh, delirium tremens—on the second day post surgery. This is now his fifth day here in the ICU, and we are slowly weaning him off the respirator." The resident stopped and turned to see if there were any questions.

One of the junior residents chimed up, "Was he much of a drinker prior to his accident?"

"According to the family, he drank alcohol every night but they really didn't know how much. His blood alcohol on admission was 0.22, which is obviously well over the legal limit. At that level, even chronic drinkers like Mr. Payne are clearly impaired and should not be driving."

Dr. Williams spoke up next, "Almost eighty percent of the patients that we see here in the ICU are here with some problem related to alcohol abuse. It could be GI bleeding, an auto accident caused by alcohol, pancreatitis, or numerous other health problems clearly related to ETOH abuse—including domestic abuse. It's a major health problem in the U.S. that's clearly not diagnosed in many cases. All physicians should always ask our patients about their use of alcohol when we take a medical history, and be highly suspicious, regardless of the answer."

Dr. Ober joined the discussion at that point. "Our experience is the same when it comes to alcohol use in our patients. We also see a high incidence of DT's in our post-op and ICU patients as well. Students, DT's occur in patients who drink heavily and then are withdrawn from alcohol 'cold turkey.' It's a real problem because the patients often deny any extensive use of alcohol prior to being admitted but then suddenly develop post-op complications that keep them in the hospital longer, or make their underlying condition far worse.

"I feel that I need also to comment on the presentation made by the resident. There's no doubt that this man was very stupid in not wearing his seatbelt but we don't need to make snide comments about this in our presentation. As the lawyers like to say 'res ipse loquitor' or 'the thing speaks for itself.' It's always amazing to me how many people don't wear seatbelts despite all the public education on the subject. The ER doctors can tell you story after story of terrible accidents in which people survived because they wore their seatbelts, and others were killed because they weren't wearing seatbelts and were thrown about inside the car or thrown out of the car. It's sheer stupidity, and I'll never understand why people don't use them. That gets me thinking about another somewhat similar subject. Anyone know what effect cell phone use has on your risk of auto accidents?"

The senior resident, Dr. Tom Barringer, spoke up. "I saw a *Dateline* show on this very subject the other night. In the story, they noted some research that indicated those using cell phones had a four times higher rate of accidents than those not using them. It was very scary stuff as they showed people dialing phones and then running off the road, or plowing into other cars at only 35 miles per hour. Many experts would like to ban cell phone use in cars, or at least require the use of hands-free phones, but they realize that they've got to get legislators to pass the laws first. Some cities have already banned their use. Unfortunately, the majority of politicians have never been known to be out front on the tough issues despite the overwhelming common sense they might make." The group couldn't help but laugh at that comment despite the seriousness of the subject.

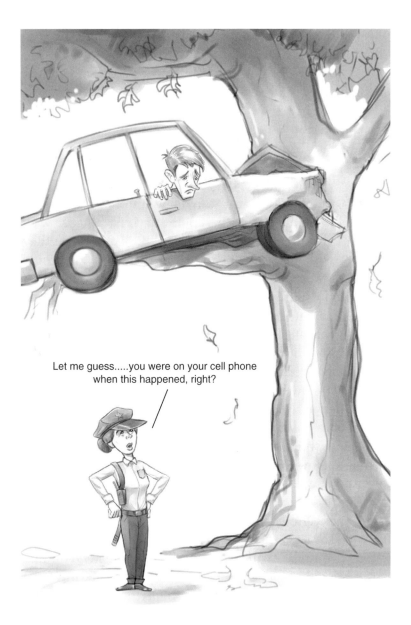

The group moved on to the next patient. Dr. Don Schumacher, the local internist caring for this patient, happened to be reviewing the chart in the room. "Dr. Schumacher, we're just making rounds and since you're here, would you mind giving us a brief rundown on your patient?" Dr. Williams asked.

"Sure, no problem. Glad to do it. Mrs. Gomez is a thirty-five-year-old Hispanic woman who developed numerous complications following a measles infection that she contracted from one of her younger daughters. She developed measles encephalitis and was admitted to the hospital. While in the hospital, Mrs. Gomez developed a nosocomial bacteremia that ended up causing a bacterial endocarditis. She is currently being treated with antibiotics for the endocarditis but she's now in congestive heart failure due to the infection on her mitral and aortic valves. We're doing all we can but as one of your fellow residents so aptly put it, she's getting the 'Will to Live Test.' It's really up to her immune system now."

Dr. Schumacher shook his head and said, "You know what I find the saddest part of this whole story? I believe all this was preventable. If her children had gotten their routine childhood immunizations, as they should have had, then it's unlikely Mrs. Gomez would have contracted either the meningitis, or its complication, the bacterial endocarditis. As a result of this tragic case, I did some research and found that the immunization rates in Hispanic children are the lowest of any group in this country. It makes no sense to me since vaccinations are free at county health departments everywhere. What a damn tragedy! So unnecessary."

Dr. Ober spoke up at that point. "That's so unnecessary and a sobering thought for us all. Maybe now's a good time for Dr. Williams and me to try our little experiment. I asked him to pull a list of the names of patients who had been in the ICU, and who are still in the hospital. What I'd like to do now is for all of us to go out and see these patients and interview them about their experiences here in the ICU. I spoke to Dr. Keith Payne at the LSU-Shreveport School of Medicine the other day, and he told me he's done this same little experiment with his medical team with great success. It made sense to me because not only do about 50% of ICU patients die on us despite our best efforts, but also many of the patients that we see never get to speak to us because they're always on a ventilator. The other thing—we rarely, if ever, get to see our ICU patients after they leave us, so we never get to really appreciate our success stories. It's hard for us to remember the ultimate good that we do when we're always up to our elbows in sick patients. It can be so discouraging and overwhelming at times. We need to be able to put a personal face on the severely ill patient we care for. It's the reason we do what we do."

Dr. Williams and Dr. Ober then led the group out of the ICU and down to the opposite end of the hall to one of the other rooms on the general medical floor. Dr. Williams knocked and the group entered the room. "Mr. Towsey, I'm Dr. Williams, the attending in the ICU, and this is Dr. Ober, a visiting professor who is here sharing his knowledge with us today. The remainder of this bedraggled group of misfits behind me is this month's medical team. We came by to visit you to see how you've been doing since you left our ICU. We were able to speak to you but we couldn't hear your side of things while you were in the ICU."

Mr. Towsey beamed a huge smile. "Thanks, Dr. Williams, I have to tell you. I owe you guys my life. My family tells me that I was pretty damn sick, and that I almost didn't make it. I'm afraid that I don't remember any of my stay in the hospital until I got here in my room. It's like an empty space in my life. I only know it happened to me because my family told me all about it. It's a good thing you got me today since I'm supposed to leave for home tomorrow."

"Bet you're looking forward to that since you've been in the hospital for almost six weeks?"

"I've got three beautiful grandchildren, two great kids and a wonderful wife, so the answer to your question is a huge 'Yes.' I'm really looking forward to going home. Thanks to you guys, I've been given a new lease on life. I'm not ready to leave this life yet. I know that I'll have to work hard to make some health changes in my life." The emotion in his voice was obvious and it touched the whole group.

After a few more brief exchanges, the group left Mr. Towsey and proceeded to visit five more patients who had been in the ICU previously. Some would not be going home right away, some would have a long stay in rehab and some would ultimately die due to further complications of their underlying problems but they all expressed an overwhelming gratefulness and appreciation for the care they had been given and for a second chance at life. The residents and students came away with a very personal appreciation of how their hard work made a difference in the lives of their patients and their families. It was a part of medicine that many of them had rarely gotten a chance to see.

✣ Perspectives for Doctors ✣

Medical students are taught how to diagnose, how to cure, how to prevent disease, and how to prolong life. What they are not taught is how to deal with dying patients. Medical education appears to be skirting end-of-life care issues. In 1995, only 26% of residency programs in the U.S. offered a course in end-of-life care in their curricula while information on the subject was absent in nearly 57% of the fifty top-selling textbooks from multiple specialties. Many medical schools have one or two lectures on death and dying that cover the five stages of dying but do little to address terminally ill patients' needs.

What's missing from the curricula is the hands-on learning required to deal with the unexpected emotions of the patients and of the doctors themselves. Students need to be prepared to deliver a terminal diagnosis and to conduct a family meeting about the diagnosis or the death of a patient. Dr. Kirsti Dyer, a primary care doctor in California, has stated, "How you tell a family that their loved one died can have a significant impact on their grief response."

Delivering good end-of-life care requires good communication skills. Physicians need to pay close attention to the words they use, the setting in which to give bad news, and the attitude with which they approach the subject. They need to be prepared and anticipate how the patient and/or the family will respond to the news. They need to understand cultural and religious differences as well. The bottom line: Medical education has failed to prepare physicians for end-of-life issues.

Too often physicians and students are taught only how to deal with their patients' physical needs, and never learn how to be consolers and comforters. Many physicians believe that this is the role of nurses, social workers and clergy. Prior to the advances of twentieth-century medicine, solace and comfort were about all previous generations of physicians had to offer their patients. With all the medicine and technology that physicians have at their disposal today, the death of a patient is often viewed as a personal failure. Medical schools promote the image of doctor-as-savior.

In 1997 the Institute of Medicine appointed the Committee on Care at the End of Life. That group quickly recommended that health professionals initiate changes in education to improve physicians' ability to care well for dying patients. The Robert Wood Johnson Foundation gave almost $1,000,000 to the Medical College of Wisconsin to develop and provide end-of-life care educational requirements and materials to teaching faculty, continuing education directors and curricular deans. With the aging of the Baby Boomer population, doctors will be dealing with death and dying issues in unprecedented numbers in the future.

The hospice movement is one of the best-known end-of-life support organizations and has done more than almost any other organization to support terminally ill patients and their families. The hospice philosophy is to provide support and services to enable individuals to live their remaining days with grace and dignity and to die peacefully. The focus of hospice care is on individual autonomy and quality of life. They offer expert advice on pain management and symptom control as well as psychosocial and spiritual care to terminally ill patients and their family.

The key for all of us, whether we are doctors or patients, is education. Patients shouldn't depend totally on their doctors, and the more educated we can al become about the various options, including the support groups that are available, the easier it will be to obtain the care patients need . . . and deserve.

Questions for Patients to Ask When Faced with a Serious Diagnosis

1. What can I do to help myself cope with my diagnosis?
2. Where can I get more information about my problem?
3. Are there support groups or self-help groups that may provide additional information or support?
4. Are there other patients of yours with a similar diagnosis that I might speak to who could help me?
5. Are there "alternative" medicine approaches that might help with my problem?

10

Pediatrics—Children Are Not Just Little Adults

"The secret of genius is to carry the spirit of the child into old age."

–Aldous Huxley

The Advisor finished putting his food on the tray and walked to the cafeteria's checkout line. While standing in line, he looked for an open table so that he could sit and eat rather than taking the food back to his office. The cafeteria was mobbed with people in scrubs and white coats as well as patients and family members. Halfway across the cafeteria he spied the Student with some other young people dressed in white lab coats. He guessed that they were all classmates so he decided to sit with them and see how things were going.

"Mind if I join you all?" he asked as he sat.

"Sure. No problem," replied one of the female students.

"Great," said another.

"Uh, no, sir . . . but we were just about ready to leave and I don't want you to have to eat by yourself," replied the Student somewhat reluctantly.

The Advisor pretended not to notice the less than enthusiastic welcome by his advisee.

"Are you all in my Student's same class in medical school?" he inquired of the group as he sat down.

"Yes, sir," answered one of the female med students. "We all just started our Pediatrics rotation."

"How's it been so far?" the Advisor asked, trying to draw them out.

One of the students who looked like he was young enough to still be in grade school spoke right up, "I hate to admit it but it's really scary. Most of the patients can't tell you what's wrong and all they seem to do is cry when you get near them. I get so nervous when I examine these kids because the mothers are right there and I'm afraid they're thinking that I'm doing something to hurt their little one. It hasn't been any fun up to this point and I don't see it getting any better."

The Advisor smiled knowingly before answering, "That sure brings back some painful memories of my own first experience on pediatrics, even these many years later. I certainly agree that it can be really frustrating. Mind if I share some things that I've learned over the years that might help you?"

All the other students immediately nodded their enthusiastic approval while the Student just rolled his eyes.

What is he going to say now? I hope that he won't go off on one of his touchy-feely tangents. If he does that, we could be here forever.

"There are two simple rules to remember that have *always* served me well when taking care of children. I learned them from my old mentor, Dr. Jerry Schiebler, the chief of Pediatrics at the University of Florida. They've saved me from missing a diagnosis many a time, and I hope they'll help you just as much, no matter what your ultimate specialty is.

"Rule #1—If a mother tells you that her child is sick or not acting normally, believe her until proven otherwise.

"Do any of you have children?" the Advisor asked the students.

They all shook their heads to indicate no.

"Well then, let me explain Rule #1 in a little more depth. Mothers generally know their children better than anyone else in the world. This is no slight to fathers but, in our society, the role of caring for children generally falls to mothers. They know when their child is not himself or herself, even when that child appears normal to an uninformed observer. If you don't pay attention to the mother, father or caretaker who brings that child to you, you'll miss an important clue, and **you will get burned.** Young children can't tell you what or how they're feeling so you have to use their mothers, or their primary caregivers, as your eyes and ears. You'll never go wrong if you do that."

The Advisor looked at the group to ensure their interest and then continued, "With children, especially the younger ones, there is less margin for error in delaying care than in adults. For example, a child with meningitis can go downhill in a real hurry and suffer permanent disabilities if not treated early enough, while adults can usually tolerate a bit more delay. They can also provide you with more information but only if you're smart enough to ask the right questions. Make sense?"

He saw a number of heads nod in agreement, so he continued.

"Rule #2—Sick kids look sick.

"I know it sounds simple but since kids can't or won't speak to you, you have to learn to read their body language. It will always tell you how sick they really are."

The Advisor stopped for a few seconds before continuing. "Let me put this into perspective for you. How does each of you act when you're sick?"

One of the female students immediately responded, "I don't feel like doing anything. I lie around and just want to

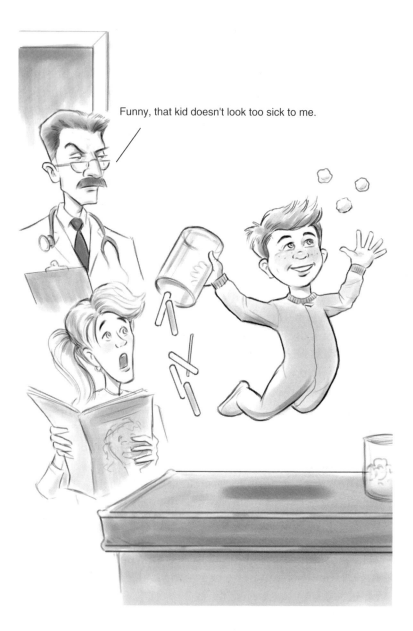

be left alone. I usually feel so miserable that being around people is a real chore and being nice is virtually impossible. It's like I want to be left alone to die . . . or get better. Sometimes I don't even care which one."

"Beautiful!" exclaimed the Advisor. "That's my point exactly. A baby can't express him or herself but only wants to be left alone. Babies don't understand why they feel miserable. Sometimes they just want to be held by the person that they identify comfort and warmth with—usually their mothers—and sometimes even that doesn't work. They don't feel like playing, and nothing will satisfy them. They lie around like you would and that's exactly what you need to look for in these children. They just don't have that sparkle in their eyes. The bottom line: if you use your senses, pay attention to your gut, and listen to what the person who cares for the baby says, you'll never go wrong."

The Advisor looked at the group to check out their level of interest before continuing. "Look, let me ask you. What's the worst thing that could happen if you think something just isn't right with a child and you decide to do a more in-depth workup?"

With some obvious reluctance, one of the students ventured an answer, "Well, testing isn't without risk and there is a cost attached."

"You're exactly right," the Advisor replied, "but neither of those things are really that bad when you consider the alternative of a missed diagnosis. Most testing has very little risk attached to it and the cost is minimal when it comes to someone's health. Sure there's the extra time spent in the ER or the doctor's office, but the family feels better because they know you are really being thorough and that you hear their concern for their child. Basically, there is no real downside to doing a more complete evaluation."

One of the students squirmed in her seat, coughed and then asked, "Sir, have you ever had a bad experience when taking care of kids? I mean . . . have you ever not followed your intuition and you regretted it later?"

The Advisor smiled ruefully before answering. "That's a good, fair and brave question. No, I personally haven't been hurt by not following my gut instinct but let me tell you about someone who was. When I was a resident on pediatric surgery, one of my fellow residents missed something that he says still haunts him to this day. Here's the story. My friend was called to the ER one night to evaluate a little two-year-old girl who was brought in by her mother who told him that her child just wasn't acting like herself. When my friend went in to examine her, the child was acting fairly normally but had a temperature of 101.5 degrees. He did a basic exam but only noted a runny nose on the chart. The mother explained that she had given the child some pediatric Motrin about an hour earlier and that the child had been lying around for the last several hours. She was concerned and wanted her thoroughly checked out. My fellow resident didn't really listen to what she said and did nothing except to briefly examine the little girl. He told the mother that her daughter had a simple cold, to treat her symptoms and her fever, and to follow-up with her doctor the next day or the day after." The Advisor stopped to take a bite of his sandwich.

"Don't stop now," one of the med students implored. "What happened next and what's still haunting him?"

The Advisor chewed a bit more before continuing, "The mother took her child home but by the next morning her daughter was more moribund and her temp wasn't controlled by the various anti-pyretics. Because of that, the mother brought her back to the ER right away. She was examined by another doctor who ordered a CBC, urinalysis, and a spinal tap. The little girl was found to have bacterial meningitis and now has permanent brain damage because she wasn't treated soon enough. Who will ever know what might have happened to her if she had been diagnosed the evening before? Maybe nothing . . . or maybe everything. Either way, my friend will live with the memory of this little girl for the rest of his life. He confessed to me later that in retrospect, he probably had treated the mother's complaints more cavalierly than he should. He'd been up for almost twenty-four hours and was tired and hadn't really listened to what the mother had said. He hated that he hadn't done a few more tests or taken more time with the mother and her daughter but he just didn't. It was tragic for everyone concerned."

The Advisor could see that his story had had a very sobering effect on the group. This was good if it helped them take care of their pediatric patients with more care in the future. The Advisor then took an article from his bag and handed it to the Student.

"Here's an article that I think may be useful for all of you as well. I've got a few copies because I've just come from a meeting with Dr. John Nackashi, the head of ambulatory pediatrics at the University of Florida, who gave me the article. Dr. Nackashi is a most interesting guy, as is his whole family. He is one of this country's leading advocates for children with disabilities or those with special needs. He and his wife have traveled all over the world helping children with cleft palates get the care they need.

"He and his family put together a booklet to help the parents of children with special needs obtain the help they need from federal and stage agencies. These problems can be overwhelming and it's nice to know where to go for support and help. His wife illustrated the book and his two sons have put together a CD-ROM program with music they've written to further help families deal with these issues. When we met we reviewed some materials various parents of children with special needs had written to help healthcare providers do a better job of understanding their needs." The

Advisor stopped and asked, "Is this of interest to you or should I stop?"

All the other med students nodded their heads to indicate their interest.

"As with many things in medicine and in business, we need to learn to listen to those actually receiving the service. They often have the greatest insight into where the problems lie and what changes can improve the care for the average person receiving the care. Computer software companies have learned that if they use beta testing with small groups of users prior to the full release, they have software that is much more user-friendly, plus they have fewer complaints. Businesses that implement quality improvement programs have found that employees who are involved in a particular process commonly provide innovative suggestions that improve efficiency and save costs. When emergency rooms began implementing non-urgent care areas of the ER to handle non-emergent medical problems, they noted big decreases in waiting time for these problems and less frustration on the part of those being served. Make sense?

"Of course it does, but why don't we do more innovative things to improve the service we provide to patients? Why don't we 'listen more to our customers,' to use a business term?

"To be blunt, because we're stupid. First, healthcare professionals are like anyone else when it comes to change. Real change always knocks people out of their comfort zone and is always stressful. They think, 'The old way is working just fine so let's not change things and get everyone upset.' Second, healthcare professionals suffer from the NIH or 'not invented here' syndrome. It can't be that good if they didn't think of it. Third and finally, physicians can be arrogant. Because they are very smart people, they think they can do everything well. That's just not the case, especially when it comes to running their offices. They don't hear the complaints like their staff does so they assume everything is wonderful. They don't feel like they have to listen to anyone else."

Dr. Stephanie Richter, one of the Pediatric attendings, approached the table and with a stern look on her face, said, "So this is where you all have been hiding." When the students turned to her, she broke into a big grin. "You know we have the outpatient clinic that started five minutes ago, and you all have been missed. I thought I saw you sitting here when I was eating earlier so I thought I'd come back and retrieve you from the old windbag here."

The Advisor laughed heartily at that last remark before replying, "I've been duly and rightfully chastised by one of my former students. Get out of here all of you before I get into even more trouble." The students got up quickly and followed Dr. Richter to the ambulatory pediatrics area of the ER. The hospital had learned from past mistakes that pediatric patients in the ER needed to be seen by those used to dealing with their unique problems, much like surgery patients or geriatric patients.

Dr. Richter picked up a chart, scanned it, and then queried the group, "What's the leading cause of death in children between the ages of one and eighteen?"

"Infections?" answered one.

"Wrong, not even among the top five, believe it or not, but thanks for playing, contestant number one."

"Cancer?" guessed another student.

"Getting warmer. Better luck next time, contestant number two. Now for our final player."

The Student knew he was on the spot but for some reason wasn't flustered. "Accidents," he blurted out with conviction.

"Excellent! Our last contestant has just won $10,000. Accidents or unintentional injuries are the leading cause of death in this age group and far exceed all others. The sad part is that so many of these deaths are preventable by just using good common sense, like keeping medicines or household cleaners out of the reach of children, using infant car seats properly, or watching children around pools. It gets me so angry because there is nothing harder or worse for me than having to tell a parent that his or her child is dead. It's something I hope none of you ever have to do in your career as a physician."

They then entered the room and quickly saw why Dr. Richter had asked the question. The patient was a two-year-old child with a huge hematoma of her right forehead and a large abrasion on her face and right arm. She had fallen from a shopping cart in the nearby supermarket because her mother had failed to secure her in her seat using the safety strap. It was a totally preventable accident that could have had serious consequences, such as skull fracture or hemorrhage in the brain. Dr. Richter had already worked the child up thoroughly and luckily found no major problems. After a serious conversation with the mother about preventing injuries in her child, she let them leave with some warning signs to watch for in the next twenty-four to forty-eight hours.

Before moving on to the next patient, Dr. Richter asked another question, "What's the third leading cause of death in young people between the ages of one and twenty-four? Before you answer, contestants, there's only one answer allowed for your team here in the final round of our quiz. Please huddle your team, Student, and give me your best guess. The clock is ticking."

The students quickly put their heads together and after a lively discussion answered, "Cancer is the third leading cause of death."

"An excellent guess but wrong. The answer is homicide, followed very closely by suicide in those ten to twenty-four.

It's pretty sad to think that children in the United States die from these causes. I can see Bosnia, the Middle East, or Ethiopia with problems like these, but here? For the most part, many of us lead such protected lives that we have no idea this is an issue. You can walk two miles down the street here in this city and it becomes a very real fact of life. It's like a war zone at times, including the sound of sporadic gunshots. As pediatricians or doctors caring for young people, we should be some of the most active people trying to protect the children we care for. I may seem to make light by the way I ask the questions but it's only to keep myself from being too depressed about what is being done to our kids."

The group was somber when it entered the next room to see a little boy who was almost eighteen months old. His mother had brought him in because of a runny nose and a fever. Dr. Richter put the boy on the carpeted section of the floor and let him play while she spoke to the mother. She put some blocks down in front of him along with a rubber ball. She then picked the boy up and did her exam. When she was done, she turned to the mother and told her that she'd be back in a minute to discuss a treatment plan for her child.

Outside the room, she began questioning the group immediately, "What very important things did you notice about that baby and why am I concerned?"

The students mentioned his smile, his weight, his interaction with people and even his cry but none of these answers got her approval. Dr. Richter continued, "The child isn't walking and should be doing so easily by this time. He's also very slow at even pulling himself up to a standing position. He doesn't even stack blocks to any level at this time either. He's definitely behind developmentally and we need to understand why. Here's my key message to you. Developmental milestones need to be assessed at *every* encounter with children. It's one of the early warning signs that something might be amiss in a child. Don't miss that opportunity. Questions, anyone?

"Yes, Dr. Keller. Are these developmental milestones pretty rigid?"

"No, there are obviously variations between children. Some children walk at ten months and others at fifteen months, but they shouldn't be way out of line like the last child we saw is. Dr. T. Berry Brazelton at Harvard Medical School has written a book that details his child development *Touchpoints* model. His *Touchpoints* are like a map of child development that can be identified and anticipated. Parents can also get involved in supporting developmental growth by taking specific actions at each stage of development."

Dr. Richter led the group back into the examining room to see the mother and child so that she could provide information on how to treat the child's viral infection. She also explained the need for scheduling a visit to see one of the child development specialists later in the week to assess the developmental delay. The students had gained a number of different perspectives that day that would help them for a lifetime.

✦ *Perspectives for Doctors* ✦

Observing developmental milestones in young children is one of the most important things that any doctor should do while caring for them. ER doctors should observe these milestones as well because many families use the ER as their primary contact with the medical system. I picked up many developmental delays during my years in the ER and I hope that sending those patients for further evaluation may have helped in the future. If developmental milestones are not met, it can be an early indication that there are problems with the child's physical, emotional or social development.

Awareness of Dr. Brazelton's model for specific developmental *Touchpoints* and strategies for dealing with them can be useful in helping families reduce patterns of negative behavior that might otherwise result in problems in areas such as sleeping, feeding, or toilet training.

Dr. David Sacher, the Surgeon General of the United States, issued a report in 2001 focusing on the effects of violence on our children. As was mentioned, homicide is the third leading cause of death in young people between the ages of one and eighteen and the second leading cause of death in fifteen- to twenty-four-year-olds. In African-Americans, it becomes the number one reason for death. The data clearly say something horrible about our society when this is allowed to happen. Working to reduce violence is a goal worthy of any specialty group but especially important for those working with children. The violence seen on television programs, movies and cartoons can have a deleterious impact on our children. It must be stopped. We, as a profession and as individuals, must take a stand.

Dr. John Nackashi has long been a leading advocate for and supporter of the American Academy of Pediatrics (AAP) and the Maternal and Child Health Bureau's approach to providing care for patients and families with special needs and creating a "medical home" for pediatric patients.

A medical home is not a building, house or hospital, but rather an approach to providing healthcare services in a high-quality and cost-effective manner. Pediatricians, family doctors, families and allied healthcare professionals act as partners in a medical home to identify and access all the medical and non-medical services needed to help children and their families achieve their maximum potential.

Benefits of a medical home include increased patient, family, and professional satisfaction; improved coordination of care; efficient use of limited resources; and increased wellness because of comprehensive care. It must be accessible, family-centered, comprehensive, coordinated, compassion-ate and culturally competent. These are easy things to say but not always easy to deliver.

Being accessible means financially, personally and geo-graphically. Family-centered care requires recognizing that the family is the constant for the child and that there is a significant diversity among families as well as varying strengths. Continuous implies being there during transition times and critical events. It needs to be comprehensive in scope and include health promotion, injury prevention, acute and chronic illness, primary care and tertiary health-care needs. Information must be shared freely and commu-nicated to all caring for the family in a collaborative fashion. Compassionate care requires listening, assuring linguistic and cultural sensitivity and identifying family priorities and concerns.

"Children with Special Health Care Needs are those who have or are at increased risk for a chronic physical, devel-opmental, behavioral or emotional condition and who also require health and related services of a type or amount be-yond that required by children generally" (Maternal and Child Health '95). This definition can include a great many children and a wide variety of families.

"Families are the cornerstone on which pediatric care is built . . . families can be big, small, extended, nuclear, multi-generational, with one parent, two parents and grandpar-ents. We become part of a family by birth, adoption, mar-riage, or from a desire for mutual support . . . A family is a culture unto itself, with different values and unique ways of realizing its dreams" (Family Voices It's only when we treat patients in the context of family and establishing a medical home that we can begin to have a real impact on reducing the risk of long-term health problems in at-risk populations.

Finally, in November 2000, the *Archives of Pediatric Ado-lescent Medicine* had a couple of articles highlighting concerns with the training given to pediatric residents. An article by Trainor and Krug highlighted the need for further training in pediatric emergency medicine. The other by Bartel and colleagues emphasized the importance of psychosocial and communication skills, including a family-sensitive and team approach as essential parts of any good program.

Perhaps the editorial contained in this same issue sums it up best: **"As physicians, we are allowed the incredible opportunity, often within minutes of first encounter, to enter into people's lives in ways that would never be afforded to close friends or even family in a lifetime. We are allowed access to their deepest fears, insecurities, and secrets. With this privilege comes the burden of responsibility. Mastery of the broad spectrum of knowledge, skills, and attitudes necessary to accurately and compassionately perform our role defines what it means to truly be a physician and not just a technician."**

Need I say more—a statement and goal worthy of any specialty.

11

Parents, Aging and the "Sandwich Generation"

"Do not go gentle into that good night.
Old age should burn and rave at close of day.
Rage, rage against the dying of the light."

–Dylan Thomas

"It's no longer a question of staying healthy. It's a question of
finding a sickness you like."

–Jackie Mason

If it hadn't been for the millions of Baby Boomers getting older, the Student knew that he wouldn't be taking Geriatrics. Now, everyone in the medical school had to spend some time learning about older patients. The Student wasn't sure he saw the need for it because he hadn't had a lot of contact with older people, didn't ever really want to, and didn't expect much need to learn more, due to his chosen specialty.

Despite his personal feeling on the subject, the Student still found himself stuck in the hospital on a beautiful spring afternoon reviewing the chart of a patient that he had to present at rounds the next morning. It seemed like his lady had every disease known to man. She was a seventy-five-year-old woman who had diabetes, rheumatoid arthritis, heart failure, and was in remission from leukemia. She had been in and out of the hospital for years and had seen and helped train numerous doctors. Her four charts seemed to weigh almost more than he did.

How am I ever going to wade through these monstrous charts, even if they are a testament to the miracles of modern medicine? How and why does she keep on living? What keeps her going? Just ease me out if I ever get this way. You'll never get an argument from me.

The Student almost jumped out of his chair when one of the floor nurses touched him on the shoulder. "Excuse me, I didn't mean to scare you, but Dr. Hill's office just called and he'd like to see you in his office as soon as possible."

"Whoa, whoa. What do you mean Dr. Hill wants to see me in his office right away? Are you sure he meant me? Did he say why? Did he sound mad?" the Student questioned the nurse in rapid-fire fashion.

"Hey, slow down, wild man. Don't shoot the messenger. His secretary called and asked me to find you and get you to his office ASAP. That's all I know. She just said it was important and to find you now."

The Student was visibly shaken. He dumped the charts haphazardly on the desk and slowly started down to the dean's office. Dr. Hugh "Smiley" Hill had been the Dean of Students at the medical school since it began over thirty years ago and was a favorite of every medical school class. On the first day of medical school, he prided himself on being able to know the name of every student in the class, based on the picture from his or her medical school application. He was a witty, gregarious man who always had a funny story to tell. Even if the story wasn't funny, his laugh was infectious and you found yourself laughing anyway. He'd been honored with a huge roast and party on his thirtieth anniversary in the job. What had surprised many who were present were the heartfelt tributes by student after student whom he had helped behind the scenes in many special ways. Without him, many stated that they would never have made it through medical school.

What could Smiley want? I haven't done anything. I've done pretty well on all my rotations, and no one's complained as far as I know. Sure I've told a few non-PC jokes but who hasn't. Crap, I'm here now and I've still got no clue. Well, time to face the music.

"Hi, Dr. Hill. How's it going?" the Student said nervously.

Dr. Hill was born and raised in North Carolina and had a true Southern drawl that made everyone smile just hearing it. "Great, thanks. I'm sorry that I had to call you down here like I did but I thought it was fairly important to get in touch with you as soon as I could. I don't know how to say it except to get directly to the point. Your mother had a stroke today and she's now in the ICU in the hospital near your parents' home in Richmond. Your Dad called and asked me to find you, and let you know as soon as possible. He said that she was walking toward him in the living room when she suddenly keeled over and fell on her side. She couldn't speak and began to drool from where her mouth had begun to droop. The rescue squad came right away and they got her to the hospital in less than an hour. Your Dad is there with her now."

The Student was stunned. He never in his wildest dreams ever imagined that this would be why he would be called to the dean's office. "My mom's only fifty-five. How could that be? She was so healthy. She walked every day. Sure, she took some blood pressure medicine but her pressure wasn't a problem. I just don't understand it."

The Dr. Hill just let the Student talk without interruption. He realized that the Student was deeply shaken and that the news had clearly stunned him. After about fifteen minutes, the Student left Dr. Hill in a daze to contact his father and to find out what he could do to help.

After getting in touch with his dad, the Student knew that he'd better get home to his parents as soon as he could. It didn't sound good for his mother. He was able to make arrangements to fly home early the next morning. As soon as he landed, he headed directly to the hospital and was immediately directed to the ICU. He found his father sitting in a chair in the waiting room. He was shocked—it looked like he'd aged ten years almost overnight. He quickly learned from his father that his mother was doing somewhat better but still hadn't gotten the use of her left arm back, and that her face still drooped slightly on the right.

The Student knocked on the ICU door and quickly explained to the nurse who came to the door that he was there to see his mother. He was ushered to her room. The sight of his mother lying on the bed with an IV in her arm, nasal prongs for oxygen, and numerous physiologic monitors almost took his breath away. He'd never felt so helpless before. For the first time, he had a glimpse of what family members of patients he'd cared for must have felt when their loved ones were seriously ill in a hospital bed. He'd never really thought much about how other people felt when they came to see their loved ones in the hospital after surgery or after suffering some major catastrophe like a stroke or heart attack. It clearly rocked him and it would serve as a huge wake-up call that he'd be forced to think about later on.

His mother couldn't speak to him because she was sleeping but he could plainly see the drooping of the right side of her face secondary to the stroke. Fortunately for his mother, she'd made it to the hospital in less than an hour and had gotten treated for her stroke within two hours. The Student knew that to have the best chance of reversing the blockage that often causes a stroke, the medicine had to be given within three hours—and ideally, the sooner the better to reduce the risk of the anti-thrombolytic's side effects. These "golden few hours" for treatment could sometimes reverse the symptoms of the stroke and reduce the resulting disability. He couldn't tell at this point whether or not his mother had gotten any benefit from the medicine.

He sat in the corner of the ICU room just watching his mother until the relative silence was interrupted by a group of seven doctors entering the room. He knew from his medical school experience that this was obviously morning rounds. None of the doctors bothered to introduce themselves to him but simply asked him to leave the room until they were finished.

"This is my mother and I just flew in from . . ."

"Son, I don't care who you are at the moment. We've got work to do and we only have a limited amount of time so could you please leave <u>now</u>," uttered the senior member of the group. He immediately turned back to the group and started to look at the chart by the bed.

"But, you don't understand, I'm in . . ." the Student started to say.

The next man in line quickly interrupted before the Student could tell the doctors that he was in medical school and that he wouldn't get in the way. "I guess you didn't hear what was said. You need to leave now. We've got a job to do here. We know what's best for the patient. Nurse, please escort this young man from the room now."

The Student was stunned as he was escorted from the room. *Why won't they listen to what I'm trying to say? They won't even let me finish! They're just so rude and cold. They didn't even introduce themselves. Don't they understand that this is my mother and I know her better than they could ever hope to?*

My father and I certainly know what my mother's wishes would be. I can't believe this is happening. I don't think any of my teachers would do anything like this. This is no way to treat people.

The Student slowly sat down next to his father when he got back to the ICU's waiting room. He was pale and clearly was shaken by the way he had been treated.

"What happened, son? You look like you've seen a ghost. Is your mother all right?" his father asked with great concern. "Did seeing your mother like that upset you that much? I know she didn't look good, but the nurses tell me that she seems to be improving."

The Student just stared dazedly toward some spot on the wall for a minute before replying. He shook his head and said, "Dad, it was awful how Mom looked but I'm somewhat used to seeing sick people. I know in my gut that Mom's chances are really good since she's basically very healthy, and she got to the hospital so soon. What got me so upset is the way the doctors just treated me when I was in Mom's room. They were rude and wouldn't even listen to a thing I was saying. I felt so frustrated because they wouldn't listen to anything I tried to say. I wouldn't treat a dog the way they just treated me." The Student stopped for a few seconds before continuing, "How have they treated you when you talked to them?"

His father uttered a small laugh, "Oh, I've never spoken to the doctors. I've gotten all the information about your mom's condition from the nurses taking care of her. They told me that it was the policy of the doctors in the ICU to let them act as liaisons with the families. You have to understand, son. The doctors here are extremely busy and like to spend their time with the patients doing whatever testing that's needed and not with their patients' families. I didn't want to upset them so I went along with the way things work here, plus I thought you could more easily speak to them . . . and then explain things to me."

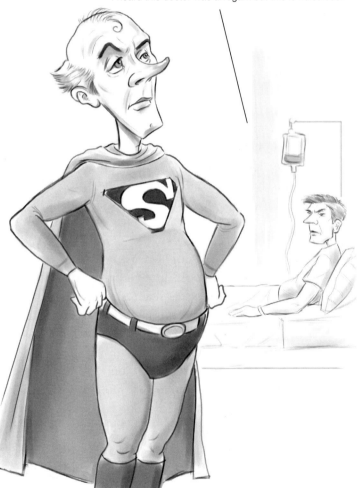

The Student was again stunned. He couldn't believe what he was hearing. It was so different from the way he had learned to do things at his medical school. He hadn't thought much about what his teachers were saying until now. It all began to make some sense. He could finally see how frustrating poor communication could be, and how angry it could make family members . . . and he'd only experienced a couple minutes of it.

The Student was really angry at this point but didn't want to get his father upset. He knew if he raised a ruckus right now that his father would worry that the doctors might not do all that they could for his mother. He also knew that his father didn't want to get branded as one of those "difficult" family members that no one wanted to deal with. Instead, the Student decided to talk to the head nurse and see what she could do to improve the situation. Before he could move to the door of the ICU, one of the nurses came through the door and with a big smile on her face called his father's name.

"I've got some great news for you. Your wife is awake and wants to speak to you. It looks like getting your wife to the hospital really paid off. She's a great testament to how rapid treatment of strokes can make all the difference. She still has some weakness in her left leg but her face is back to normal again."

The Student and his father quickly entered the ICU and could instantly see that the nurse had spoken the truth. His mother was now sitting in bed at a forty-five-degree angle and looked just as pale as before, but she now had a big smile on her face. As they drew closer to her beside, she spoke quietly to them. "I guess I gave you two quite a shock, didn't I?"

His father was so overcome with emotion that all he could do was sit beside the bed, pick up his wife's hand, caress it, and then kiss it. The Student quickly spoke for them both and tried to make it as light-hearted as possible, "Dad was a little worried but I wasn't the least bit concerned because I know what a great kidder you are, plus you're a mean old bird . . . or at least that's what I remember Dad saying all the time when I was growing up. Fortunately, I just happened to have a little time off from med school and I was planning to come home anyway."

His mother just laughed. "You can't even lie well. I thought they would at least teach you new young doctors how to tell patients what they want to hear a bit more convincingly. You know TOV, tone of voice, is very important. Your heart's just not in what you're telling me. Remember your grandfather's old saying, 'You can't B.S. a B.S.-er.' So, which one of you is going to 'fess up and tell me what happened to me?"

The Student smiled but replied in a much more serious tone now, "You had a stroke. Dad said one minute you were there and the next you were down on the floor. Frankly, you scared the hell out of us. Dad and I could only think the worst while hoping for the best." The Student took a moment before continuing. "Have you had any warning signs or funny feelings in your head before this episode?"

"No, I've felt fine up to now. I've increased my vitamins of late but otherwise doing my usual routine. Frankly, I feel pretty good now except that my left hip is killing me every time I try to move it. I guess I must have fallen on it."

At that point, one of the nurses entered the room and informed everyone that visiting time was over and that her patient didn't need to be tired out and pushed too much. All agreed so the Student and his father quickly uttered their goodbyes.

The next morning the Student returned to the ICU and found his mother so improved that she was sitting up in bed and eating heartily. "Mom, how's my favorite patient doing? The way you're eating I'd have to guess that you like the hospital food better than Dad's cooking. Just don't stay in here to try and gain weight. How's your hip today?"

"I hate to complain but it's so sore that I can't get up to walk even though I feel like I'm back to my normal self."

"Did you tell your doctors about it?"

"Well, I tried to but they sort of pooh-poohed me and told me that it was just sore from my fall. You know, now that I think about it, they didn't even examine it. They seemed more concerned about my mental state. They kept asking me to remember things, count backwards, stick out my tongue and touch my finger to my nose. How strange."

"I can't believe they never even checked your leg. Do you mind if I look at it?" the Student said with great concern.

"Of course not, dear. After all you're the doctor in the family now," laughed his mother.

"Mom, I don't want to be your doctor but I am concerned about you."

The Student slowly began to move his mother's left leg. As soon as he moved it out to the side even slightly, his mother grimaced in pain. He then touched the area by the hip where it hurt the most and again his mother jumped. As he was doing this, the nurse came in and asked what he was doing. When he demonstrated the problem to the nurse, she also became concerned. Between them they decided to suggest an X-ray to the treating physician. The nurse said that she'd get that done and then come get the Student when the results were back.

A few hours later the nurse came to get the Student and his father. "I hate to tell you this but your wife has a fractured hip and will need to go to surgery tomorrow. It's no wonder she's been in pain. The other problem that needs to be addressed that was found on her X-rays is the marked osteoporosis that your wife has already. She and I spoke about the many ways that are now available to help prevent osteoporosis. She told me that neither her Ob-Gyn nor her primary care doctor had ever mentioned medicines or hormone replacement therapy to her. I'm so surprised especially since her own mother had problems with osteoporosis as well."

The Student was stunned. His thoughts were all over the place. *How in the hell could her doctors not have mentioned all the different drugs that were available to her in this day and age? The research clearly showed their advantages, albeit there are some serious side effects with hormone replacement therapy but a woman could be given choices and allowed to make that decision along with her doctor. And why did the nurse and I have to ask for the X-ray? Why didn't her doctors listen to her complaints? My mother isn't a complainer. Why won't they talk to families? They could only help them to understand their patient better. Talk about malpractice. I don't know which doctors I'm more pissed off at. This is no way to treat people. It reminds me of the story my Advisor told—Oh, Good God! This is exactly what he's been trying to get across to me about the Art of Medicine. They're treating the disease but haven't listened to the patient.* The light had gone on for the Student. The wake-up call had come and so much had suddenly become obvious. All the Art of Medicine stuff had, for the first time, begun to make sense.

"Dad, this is a crock of crap. Mom is too young to have osteoporosis as severe as she has. I've learned enough to know that it's largely preventable, thanks to various medications, vitamin D and calcium supplements but only if they're begun at the right time. I am so damned mad at her doctors. I can finally begin to understand why physicians get hit with malpractice suits."

His father tried to soothe his feelings but the Student would have no part of it. He realized that his father's generation just didn't question doctors and still kept them on a pedestal for the most part. Things would never change that way.

They both returned to the ICU and again the Student's mother had a smile on her face. "Judging from your faces, I can see that you've heard the news. At least that explains why I was such a wimp and couldn't put weight on my leg. I always associated a fractured hip with old age and I never thought of myself that way. I saw some bumper stickers in a magazine the other day that I guess I'll have to put on my car. 'Age only matters if you're cheese,' or 'Age is an issue of mind over matter. If you don't mind, it doesn't matter.' My favorite is, 'Old age and treachery will overcome youth and skill anytime.' What do you boys think?"

The Student replied with obvious anger. "Mom, this is no laughing matter. You're not old. This should never have happened. Your doctors haven't done you any favors by not giving you some choices about how to prevent osteoporosis. There are some great medicines out there that can reduce your risk of osteoporosis. You've probably seen some of the ads on TV yourself, since the drug companies are advertising directly to consumers now. Didn't you ever question your docs about this, especially since Granny had this same problem?"

"Son, I know what you're saying but they were doing the best they could. I trusted them. You have to understand, people in my generation were brought up in such a way that we rarely questioned authority figures. I'm just not used to questioning my doctors—plus they're always so busy. I sometimes feel like I'm imposing at times. After all, my problems aren't life-threatening."

"Mom, one of the things I'm learning in medical school is that doctors need to find the time to listen. They need to know their patients, and they need to ask questions to find out what their patients' needs are. On the other side, I'm also learning that patients need to get more involved in their own medical care. It's a partnership and a relationship so it requires two people to make it work most effectively."

God! the Student thought, *I'm starting to sound just like my professors. If my Advisor could only hear me now, he wouldn't be-*

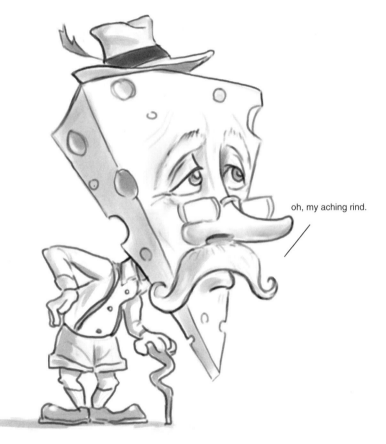

oh, my aching rind.

Age only matters if you're cheese.

197

lieve it. One thing's for certain, the way my Mom's been treated
will certainly change the way I deal with my older patients.

"Son, my parents and a lot of my generation grew up respecting doctors and we just don't question what's done.
Who were we to question people with all those years of
training?"

"I understand, Mom, but maybe that's not the best approach to medicine today. Let Dad and me go out and get a
bite while you eat. We'll be back later to see you. Love you,
Mom."

The Student left and went to the waiting room. He came
across his grandfather who had just arrived to see his oldest daughter. "Hi, Grandpop, it's great to see you!" the Student said, giving him a huge hug. "Where's Grandma?"

His grandfather looked down at the floor and sheepishly
replied almost inaudibly, "She's in a nursing home."

The Student was stunned. He had just been pole-axed by
the news. First his mother, and now this. "What do you
mean, Grandpop? I don't understand. When did this happen? Why? How come I don't know anything about it?" The
Student couldn't get the questions out fast enough in his
confusion.

His grandfather replied with some hesitation, "Your
grandmother had slowly deteriorated physically over the
last few months, thanks to a series of mini-strokes. The
strokes, along with her already existing mild dementia, also
caused a rapid decline in her mental function. It had gotten
so bad that we couldn't leave her by herself because she
couldn't be counted on to do even the simplest of things. For
instance, I came home one day after going for a walk and
she'd turned all the gas burners on and had put an empty
pot over one. The rest were bare. That same week, I found
her wandering in the backyard barefoot without a jacket
when it was forty degrees outside. She didn't know why she
was in the yard or where the house was. That's when we de-

cided to take some action. It was the hardest decision of my life, but with my heart condition, I just couldn't watch her or care for her as she needed to be." The sadness in his grandfather's voice was almost palpable and it touched the Student deeply.

"But, why didn't you tell me?"

"We didn't want to bother you with all the pressure you had on you in medical school. You work so many hours and have so little time to yourself. You didn't need another worry and besides, what could you really do?"

The Student had never felt more frustrated. He was at a loss for words and retreated inside himself for a minute so that he could find the right words to say.

"Granddad, sometimes Mom, Dad and you really make me mad . . . and this is one of those times. Don't you all know that it's never a bother with me, that we're family and we should help each other out when we're in trouble? Who better than me when it comes to medical problems? Why are all of you so damned stubborn and independent?"

His grandfather just hugged the Student at that point and then went in to see his mother but returned shortly with a smile on his face. "Your mom's doing well and that's a relief for me. You know, just because we're both older doesn't mean that I stop worrying about her. She'll always be my little girl to me."

The Student had to smile at that even though his world had just been turned upside down again. The next twenty-four hours passed by but the Student didn't remember much because the recent events had put him in such a daze. His mom was going to be discharged that day and she would recover with few problems, provided the rehab went well. He had gone to see his grandmother in the nursing home but he wasn't sure that she knew who he was for most of the time. She'd only seemed to remember the distant past and didn't even remember that he was in medical school.

He headed for the airport to return to school with a very different perspective on medicine, on what should be done with patients and on the Art of Medicine.

✤ *Perspectives for Doctors* ✤

Aging describes the temporal process of growing old and is often associated with a progressive decline in our general body function. The World Health Organization defines the **elderly** as those people between the ages of sixty-five and seventy-five. The term **old** is reserved for those between seventy-five and ninety. Those over age ninety are defined as **very old.** Thanks to the Baby Boomer generation, the numbers of those over age sixty-five will reach thirty million in the next thirty years. It's estimated that by the year 2050, people aged sixty-five and older will make up 20% of the US population, with 7% of those residing in nursing homes.

Normal aging is often subdivided into two categories—**successful aging** and **usual aging.** Successful aging is found in those persons who demonstrate minimal decline in physiological function. Such mild decline is directly related to the practice of preventive health strategies over the course of a lifetime, such as not smoking, eating sensibly, and exercising. Increased educational efforts by healthcare professionals and the media in the last couple of decades will hopefully pay huge dividends for most aging Americans in the future. Usual aging is the most common kind of aging and indicates the expected decline in kidney function, hearing, vision and other systems with time.

Life expectancy has risen dramatically in the last hundred years. It was about forty-seven years in 1900 and now approaches eighty years. With more people living longer, the current Baby Boomer generation has now become known as the "sandwich" generation, because they often find themselves sandwiched between two generations of family for which they are largely responsible. This has created a unique set of problems for those sandwiched in the middle. How can they take time away from their children and their needs to tend to aging parents or relatives who need them just as much? How can they avoid feelings of guilt that plague them when they can't do all that they'd like to do for older family members because they live in distant cities? (My parents are in their eighties and live 300 miles away. Fortunately, I have two brothers who live in the same town and help to address their needs. They and their families visit regularly, take them out for meals and address problems that our parents can no longer handle for themselves. It's a tremendous relief for my sister and me.) But what about others who are caught in similar situations and have to put parents or relatives into nursing homes or assisted living situations often against their wishes? Being part of the sandwich generation has created its own unique set of pressures and emotional issues.

There are many reasons for the increase in life span we're seeing, including prevention of disease by widespread vaccinations, improved medical care in the areas of heart disease and stroke, better treatment of cardiac and cancer risk factors and better access to medical care.

The five leading causes of death in the elderly are (in order) heart disease, cancer, chronic obstructive pulmonary disease (COPD), cerebrovascular disease or strokes and accidents. Almost all of these diseases can be prevented or mitigated by paying attention to certain risk factors related to them. For instance, COPD rarely occurs in anyone who did not smoke, so by avoiding smoking one's chances of getting this breathing disease are slim and none.

The risk factors for heart disease and stroke are similar—high blood pressure, elevated cholesterol, smoking and diabetes. These are the preventable, or controllable, risk factors. If an individual has none of these risk factors, then his or her risk of heart disease or stroke will generally be very low. Obviously, there are a couple of other major risk factors but these are not controllable. They are age and family history. If patients have a family history of early heart attacks or strokes, then they need to pay even more attention to reducing other controllable risk factors as well as keeping themselves fit with a good exercise program.

Seventy-five percent of strokes occur in patients older than age sixty-five. It is the third leading cause of death in patients over seventy-five. The annual incidence of stroke is 2% and has declined over the last twenty years, due to the better management of associated risk factors. Eighty-two percent of strokes result from infarcts or blockages in the vessels within the brain. Atheromatous plaques containing cholesterol or fat in the walls of the blood vessels cause almost all of these infarcts.

Many patients have some warning sign of a stroke prior to its manifesting itself. Between 50% and 70% of strokes are preceded by a transient ischemic attack, or TIA. TIAs mimic the signs of a stroke but usually resolve within thirty minutes. These should be viewed as serious warning signs and discussed with the patient's doctor to ensure good preventive treatment.

Another major issue for the elderly is the loss of independence that occurs when they can no longer care for themselves or no longer do things that they have been doing for most of their lives, such as driving a car, paying bills or going to the store unassisted. Being dependent on others is difficult for any of us to accept but when we're younger it's usually transient, such as following surgery or a short illness. To know that it's for the rest of your life is terribly devastating and often produces severe depression in the elderly.

The lack of independence also raises the issue of caregivers. Long-term care given by family members is a central component of our current healthcare system. Approximately twenty-five million family caregivers provide an estimated $194 billion in care annually. A recent article in the *American Family Physician* notes that family members care for 80% of patients with dementia. Persons with Alzheimer's disease account for a portion of those with dementia and now number about four million, with fourteen million expected in another twenty-five years. The number of caregivers will be rising and the number of their medical problems along with them.

Many caregivers experience anxiety, depression and a sense of isolation, as well as increased rates of morbidity and mortality. Some researchers estimate that 60% to 70% of relatives caring for demented persons have medical or psychiatric illness as a result. Therefore a major tenet of geriatric care is the need to support or bolster family members who act as caregivers. Physicians need to focus on disease but should also focus on the broader psychosocial, economic and support problems.

Finally, one of the fastest growing trends in the United States is the movement to long-term care facilities of various types. An important fact to note is that all long-term care or senior residences are not the same. There are tremendous differences in facilities based on need and lifestyles. Some provide little in the way of support while others cater to those with heavy care needs. Some have special wings for the memory impaired while others have many activities for residents. And just because a facility is expensive doesn't necessarily make it better. What makes a facility good or bad most often depends on the attitude of the staff toward their clients. Much like physicians, a caring attitude makes all the difference in how someone is cared for.

A number of books and websites can help patients in selecting a facility. The following are important points for your patients or families to consider:

1. Start planning sooner rather than later. When in an emergency, it's often too late and some bad decisions can be made.

2. Figure out what kind of help is needed now and likely to be needed in the future. The National Association of Professional Geriatric Case Managers can help in the assessment.

3. Visit as many centers or facilities as possible to understand your options. Spend as much time as possible and go at various times of the day. Consider making an unannounced visit.

4. Talk to residents, family members and staff to get their assessments of the facility. Try a few meals. Are the residents well groomed? Is there a pleasant odor about the place? How does the staff interact with residents?

5. Request a contract and have it reviewed by an attorney.

6. Check for complaints about the facility with the local Better Business Bureau or with the local Department of Social Services.

Primary care physicians should know what facilities are available in their communities, what services are provided and the strengths and weaknesses of each. It's a debt you owe your patients and their families as you care for them in the later stages of their lives.

12

Family Practice, House Calls and Hospitalists

"The practice of medicine in its broadest sense includes the whole relationship of the physician with his patient. It is an art, based to an increasing extent on the medical sciences, but comprising much that still remains outside the realm of a science."

–Dr. Francis Peabody (JAMA, 1927)

"Trust gives the doctor-patient relationship meaning, importance, and substance, in the same way that love and commitment give meaning and define the quality of spousal relationships."

–Mark Hall (NCMJ, 2001)

The Student couldn't believe it. Here he was about to spend two weeks in the foothills of West Virginia in some small town that wasn't even big enough to be worthy of a McDonald's or a Wendy's.

How did I ever get sent to Nowhere, West Virginia? It had to be some kind of practical joke dreamed up by my Advisor. Why me?

Sure this was a required rotation, but much of my class had at least gotten stationed in practices that were easily accessible to large cities. This is at least an hour's drive away from any large town worth thinking about. Shades of the movie "Deliverance," or more likely it was like Andy Griffith's old Mayberry.

His thoughts were cut short as a small sign on the side of the highway indicated his arrival into the town of Hamlin, West Virginia. He quickly came to the Hamlin Medical Clinic, the site of Dr. Robert "Bob" Walker's medical practice. Dr. Walker was an institution in the area because for many years he had been the sole source of medical care for the entire county. He was a hero to the local people and was one of the most sought-after speakers nationally on the Family Practice continuing medical education circuit. He also was a Professor in the Family Practice program 100 miles away.

Dr. Walker was a thin, sandy-haired, good looking, but somewhat shy man, with a ready smile. He liked to dress casually, which just added fuel to the fire of the picture the Student had in his head of this whole primary care experience. His Advisor had spent time practicing with Dr. Walker when they both were teaching at one of the academic medical centers and he had nothing but praise for his friend's down-home wisdom. His Advisor had told him one thing before he left, "Just keep your eyes, ears and mind open and you'll learn more about real medicine than you or your classmates will learn on all your other electives combined." The Student just knew that his Advisor was having a "senior moment" when he had made that statement but he had smiled anyway.

The Student was quickly ushered back to Dr. Walker's office by one of his nurses who seemed to talk the whole time in some sort of Southern twang. He didn't really listen because all he wanted to do was get back in his car and return to the world of "good" medicine and to his beloved radiology. The medical office was just as he expected it would be.

There were books, papers, medical magazines and patient charts everywhere without any apparent system to the catastrophe. What amused the Student more were the little knickknacks and medical-related paraphernalia tucked everywhere in the office. It was just so folksy.

Dr. Walker ambled into the office and greeted the Student with a shy smile. "Glad to see you found this place. It's a bit off the beaten path and not many people would normally think to stop here, or even to set up practice here," he said with a laugh.

Oh, you can bet on that one, the Student thought. *What in the hell have I gotten myself into?*

Walker talked with a slow drawl and in an almost apologetic manner. "It's nice that you wanted to come down here and spend some time with me. I hope you'll share some of the modern medicine you're learning in the big medical center these days with me while you're here. Got a few more patients to see before we head out for lunch. Come on with me. We'll see them together." With that he pulled himself slowly from the chair and ambled across the hall to one of the exam rooms.

Sitting on the exam table was a thirty-ish appearing woman who looked a bit down in the mouth and slightly disheveled. "Hi, Laura," was Dr. Walker's greeting as he sat in a chair next to her. "This is a medical student friend of mine who's going to spend some time with me and teach me a thing or two. So tell me, what's on your mind today?"

The young woman didn't raise her head and spoke in a sad, soft voice. "My headaches are coming back again and I just can't seem to get relief with any over-the-counter medicines. I just thought maybe you could give me something for them so that I could take care of my family."

"Are you sleeping all right?"

"Yeah, no problem once I get to sleep, and I feel like sleeping all the time."

"How's your appetite?"

"Just don't seem to have one. Food isn't appealing to me."

"I guess you don't have much energy, then."

"No, not much at all. I just feel so tired."

"Can I guess that you break out in tears for no apparent reason at times?"

"Yeah, how'd you know? Could I have those 'migratory' headaches or maybe a brain tumor?"

Dr. Walker got up and walked closer to her. He raised her head, examined her neck, looked into her eyes and asked his patient do a few other simple things. "Laura, you don't have a tumor or any of those migraine headaches. What you do have is a fairly common type of headache that I can help. One of the reasons that you have most of those other symptoms that are bothering you is because you're depressed. Sometimes the chemicals inside your head get out of balance, much like your sugar does when you have diabetes. I'm going to put you on a medicine that we sometimes use in depression that will help you and your particular symptoms. It will help get those chemicals inside your head back in balance and will make you feel a great deal better, plus get rid of your headaches." Walker reached into the exam room cabinet and pulled out two weeks' worth of samples of the antidepressant, Zoloft, and gave them to Laura. "Two things you have to promise me. Take this medicine faithfully for two weeks and then come back and see me. If you have problems before then, call me but I definitely want to see you again . . . no matter what. O.K. with you?"

"I definitely will, Dr. Walker."

"Any questions for me? Good. Now, how are your little girls?"

For the first time, the young woman seemed to perk up a bit as she spoke. After another minute or so of small talk, she left with a promise to return soon. Dr. Walker and the Student saw two more patients before stopping for lunch.

Walker had had his nurses get two box lunches for them. They walked out the back door and over to a nearby park.

"Any questions for me, Student?"

The Student thought for a minute before speaking, "That wasn't much of a workup you did on that young woman with headaches. At school they'd have ordered a CT scan of her head to rule out a brain tumor. Then, you gave her some medicines that I've never prescribed before for headaches. When I was on Neurology, they treated headaches all the time and I never heard anyone use that medicine for pain."

Dr. Walker smiled slightly before answering, "What do you think her diagnosis was?"

"Well, it was clearly headaches like you said."

"No, that was really a symptom. Her real diagnosis was depression. I asked you an unfair question, in a way. You see, I've taken care of her for years, and know her family history. She's got a husband who's an alcoholic and who left her after running up a fair amount of debt. The questions I asked her confirmed the diagnosis of depression. I had already figured that's what it was based solely on her body language. Normally, she's lively and makes good eye contact and is fun to be around. She'll be back to see me in two weeks. You'll still be here so we'll soon see if I'm right or not."

Please don't remind me that I've got four weeks here. I may have to slash my wrists before then. Who ever heard of making a diagnosis like this without a better workup? Body language? Please!

Dr. Walker took a few bites of his sandwich before continuing. "I know I don't do things the same way they would at the big medical center but I'm proud of that. I know my people and that gives me a tremendous advantage over any specialist anywhere. Another thing that I've learned over the years: there's more depression out here than we've ever been led to believe from all those scientific papers. Depression is not a psychiatric disorder alone, but about 50% of the cases are due to a chemical imbalance in the brain. Once that's corrected, people get back to normal again. It has nothing to do with their life situation or events around them, but is totally out of their control, much like diabetes. Diabetics cannot will themselves to have more insulin. They often need medicines to help them get their sugar under control. They can go to all the psychotherapy they want but until they get themselves back in balance chemically, it just won't work."

They headed back inside and saw patients for another few hours. The Student got to leave early the first day so that he could get settled into his room and that was just fine with him. The Student was surprised and amazed by how few lab tests Dr. Walker ordered as well as how much time he spent just talking to his patients. It certainly wasn't the way things were done back at the medical center.

The next day in Dr. Walker's office, the day went pretty much the same. After the office practice was done, they headed for the hospital to see all of his patients confined there. The nearest hospital was a ninety-minute drive but Dr. Walker wanted to take care of his patients himself. It wasn't easy but a recent change made this somewhat easier. The hospital had just hired a couple of hospitalists to care for the inpatients.

Hospitalists were physicians who specialized in treating patients in the hospital, which meant that they didn't have an office practice of their own. It was one of the latest trends in medicine and it made a great deal of sense. Physicians who had an office practice could not easily leave their offices to come take care of their patients in the hospital when those patients started to have problems. Hospitalists could be there twenty-four hours a day to immediately look after all hospital patients. These specialists also were skilled in the latest intensive care medical techniques that the average physician in practice often didn't have time to keep up with, due to his or her practice demands.

"Dr. Walker, do you like using physician hospitalists?" the Student asked as they entered the hospital.

"Well, I have to admit that at first I didn't like them all because I was afraid they'd come between me and my patients. After a short while, I realized that my patients were actually getting better care than I could give them by myself. I could still look in on them and provide my input into their care. If it's better for my patients, then it's better for me, and I'd better learn to adjust."

They came to the first patient's room. It was a woman in her eighties who'd fallen at home and broken her hip. Her surgery had gone very well but she was still in considerable pain. Dr. Walker walked into the room, pulled a chair next to her bed, and gently cradled her hand in his own. "Mrs. McDonough, you deserved such special care that I brought another young doctor along with me to see how you're doing. He's a medical student from out of town who's sharing some of his knowledge with me. So, tell me truthfully, how's my favorite patient doing today?"

"Ah, Dr. Walker, now. Sure enough ye must be from the auld country because you've got a bit o' the blarney about ya," she said with an unmistakable Irish brogue.

Everyone smiled at that remark and you could see her spirits brighten. "You know, Mrs. Mac, you're going to have to work hard to get that hip working well again. You'll have some pain but I want to assure you that I'll be there for you whenever you need me. You're tough so I know you can do it. When you get better, what do you want to do the most? What do you do that gives you a special feeling of happiness?"

Mrs. McDonough's face beamed as she replied, "I wants to be able to go out and play with me great grandchildren agin. Just thinkin' about them and bein' able to sit with them and color or to push the little ones in their swings. Nuthin' could give me more pleasure, Dr. W."

"Perfect, that's exactly what I want you to keep in mind as you work toward getting yourself back on your feet. Keep that dream alive in front of you and you'll get there. I promise you that." He gave her hand another squeeze and got up to go. "We've got a few other folks to see tonight but we'll be back tomorrow again. Please stay out of trouble and do what they ask you. Remember, work toward your dream and not only will you get out of here soon enough but you'll be able to walk with your great grandchildren in no time."

Dr. Walker and the Student finished seeing his other patients about 7:00 p.m. and then went to the hospital lounge for a minute before leaving. "Student, we're going to make a house call but in a little different way than was done in earlier days. We're going to use the phone. I call it the Modern House Call. What I do is call some of the patients that I've seen over the past couple of days and that I've got some concerns about. Remember Mrs. Gomez who we saw today with the cough and difficulty breathing? I'll call her to make sure she's getting some relief and to ensure that she's using her medicines properly. By calling your patients, you demonstrate your concern, head off potential trips to the ER and often avoid late night calls. If for some reason, you can't make the call, then one of your office staff should do so."

"Have you ever made the old fashioned house calls to your patient's homes?"

"Yes, I have, and I still do in selected cases. House calls do teach you a great deal about your patient's home environment and support system—or lack thereof. The problem I've found with house calls is that you have no real equipment to use if needed to help evaluate your patient. What do you think is the other big reason house calls aren't done anymore?"

The Student didn't take long to respond, "It's got to be the time factor. Doctors today already have so many demands on their time. If you add the time it takes to make house calls on top of those, it really makes it virtually impossible."

"Great, you're exactly right. My family already sees less of me than both they and I want, so I'm looking for ways to give them more time, not less. It's one of the reasons that I've used more physician extenders over the years. My nurse practitioner, Claudina Ghianni, is a godsend. She spends more time with people and is extremely thorough. The women patients feel so comfortable with her and many actually prefer her rather than me. It's not threat to me, since it's all about getting my patients the best possible care. If I didn't make smart use of my office staff, I wouldn't be able to accomplish as much as I do. They also make phone calls to patients, and that eases the burden on me as well. Speaking of all this, let's get out of here and head home. It's getting late and the family's missing me. We can finish our conversation in the car."

They got into the car and headed for home. "You know, Student, medicine has undergone dramatic changes. The paradigm has shifted but patient and physician expectations under this new system haven't been well defined. It's one reason both groups are so frustrated. In the past, the family doctor was all things to all people. He would sew people up, deliver babies, treat their heart attacks, and care for the children. In recent years, physicians have had to learn new ways of practicing their professions, especially using physician extenders. Patients have had to make this same adjustment by getting used to seeing and talking with persons other than physicians. They've also had to realize that I can't be on call twenty-four hours a day, and that I couldn't do justice to a hospital practice anymore. It's an adjustment for them as well as me."

They were quiet the rest of the way home, and after the day they had, it was nice to escape to the comfort of family life.

The next week went by in a similar fashion with the Student learning the nuances of caring for the whole person. After another day of connecting with people, he finally had to ask Dr. Walker something. "How are you able to connect with people so well?"

Dr. Walker just smiled. "My basic rule is that I treat people and not the disease. I have to connect with the person to find out how my diagnosis is affecting their total life functioning. Keeping that in mind is the key, but I do have a technique that I learned early on that might be helpful for you in your future dealing with patients. It's called the BATHE mnemonic and it's an effective and efficient technique for engaging a patient on an emotional and psychological level.

"Begin with the initial **B**ackground question: What's going on in your life?

"The next question is about **A**ffect: How do you feel about what's going on?

"Then, to what's **T**roubling you: What about the situation bothers you most?

"Assess how the patient is **H**andling it: How are you dealing with this?

"Finally, provide an **E**mpathetic statement: That must be difficult for you."

Dr. Walker leaned forward to make his point. "It's all about caring for people. This is just a technique. Every physician has to put these questions into his or her own words and use this method in a way that fits their particular personality. My style won't be right for you but it's perfect for me. You're unique so you need to find your own unique way of connecting to people."

It's like what my Advisor's been saying as well. It makes sense but I'm not sure I'll ever get comfortable with all this emotional and psychological side of caring for patients. I'd feel better just treating 'em and streeting 'em.

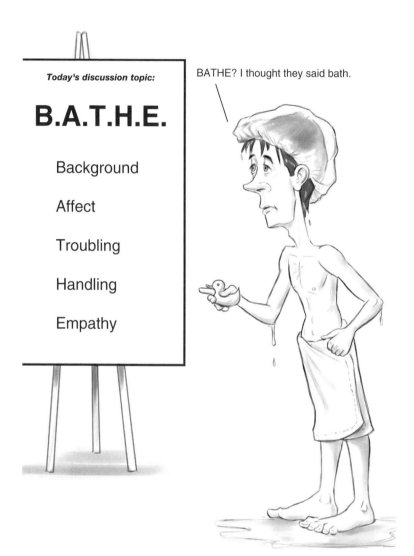

The Student had much to think about over the next couple of weeks and the time seemed to fly by, thanks to the busy days and nights. The Student even began to make some of the telephone house calls on his own with appropriate backup by Dr. Walker or his staff. A caring attitude permeated Dr. Walker's practice. The Student felt it and the patients were engulfed in it. It was such a different experience. Finally, the last day of the rotation with Dr. Walker came. The depth of the sadness that the Student felt was quite surprising and he couldn't believe that he wasn't looking forward to leaving. Dr. Walker pulled him into his office right before he was ready to leave.

"I know you'll be leaving in a few minutes to head back to school so I wanted to share some things with you. First, it's been a pleasure having you here with me for the past several weeks, and you're welcome back anytime you want to come. Second, I'd like you to seriously consider a career in Family Practice. We need more, young, bright doctors like you. You know I believe that primary care is where the action is, even though it can be extremely demanding and very tough at times. Obviously, you can make more money doing many other things in medicine, but the people rewards and emotional income in this specialty are limitless.

"If you do decide on Family Practice, I've got a few thoughts to share with you that might be helpful. Get involved in your local Family Practice department and in organized medicine in general. You need to be part of the solution and to have an impact on those medical organizations that have an influence on your professional life.

"Next, give things up only after great consideration. You will be able to do many things in your professional life but if you give up doing them or give up certain hospital privileges, it's hard to get them back again. Think about cutting back rather than cutting out.

"Stay current with CME. It's too easy not to keep up with

the latest medical advances. You can learn online but there's always something special about sharing with others in the profession in a group meeting, and no better way to learn and remember. We remember best with stories so share yours with others and they will do the same with you.

"My next point is part of the reason you're here. Keep teaching the practice of medicine. You always learn something from others as I have from you these past few weeks. Passing on knowledge to others is a way of supporting the Hippocratic Oath and is part of what we each owe to our profession—and to our patients.

"Finally, do some things that are fun for you. Remember the old saying, 'All work and no play makes Jack a dull boy.' There's a reason for that old adage. Without a hobby or some sort of recreation, it's too easy to burn out. Why do you think I play in a little band or go hiking on the weekends? Recreation is for re-creating yourself. To help remind you of the need to "recreate yourself" and because I know you're a film buff, my family and I bought you a DVD player so that you can watch some of your beloved movies. It will also help you remember us." Dr. Walker stopped, extended his hand to shake goodbye and said, "Thanks for listening. Like I said, it's been a pleasure having you here."

The Student was overwhelmed and somewhat choked up. "Dr. Walker, you've changed my life. I came here almost against my will and you opened my eyes to a part of medicine that I truly hadn't acknowledged. I won't forget you for this."

The Student shook Dr. Walker's hand warmly, got into his car and slowly headed back to the medical center deep in thought . . . and greatly confused over his career choices.

✢ *Perspectives for Doctors* ✢

The old image of the family doctor making house calls is a thing of the past. House calls have gone away because they are so cost and time-inefficient. A doctor can see five times as many patients in the office in the same time it takes to make one house call. Another disadvantage is the lack of laboratory and other equipment that might be needed to help make a diagnosis. Early in my career in medicine I would take calls at nights and on weekends. If patients sounded like they needed to see a doctor, I would often go by their homes, but two incidents made me rethink this strategy.

The first incident occurred with one of my pregnant patients. She was about thirty-seven weeks into her second pregnancy and was doing wonderfully. She had called me complaining of abdominal pain that was crampy but not regular. I asked if it could possibly be labor pains or early contractions associated with false labor. She denied that possibility. At the time I kept some basic medical equipment at home, so I told her I'd be over to see her. I went to the house, spoke to her for a few minutes, and then did a basic examination. To my great shock and dismay, she was well along in labor and was going to deliver soon. I asked her husband to call an ambulance so that we could get to the hospital as soon as possible. The ambulance came and we both headed off to the hospital together. In just a couple of minutes, I delivered a healthy baby girl in the back of the ambulance shortly before getting to the hospital. It really scared me, since the possibility of something going wrong was tremendous. I felt so helpless and out of control.

The second case involved an older gentleman who had had heart troubles in the past and was a patient of one of my fellow residents. He complained of some shortness of breath when he called. He lived nearby so I said I would come by to see him. When I got there, it didn't take me long to figure out that he was in florid congestive heart failure. He could hardly breathe because he had so much fluid in his lungs because his heart had failed. I again called an ambulance and got him admitted immediately to the hospital. He eventually made it home but that incident at his house scared me so much that I vowed to think very seriously before I ever made a house call again.

The BATHE mnemonic technique is an excellent method for connecting with patients. All of us need to feel understood and listened to, but especially when we are patients. We may not be able to cure but we can manage and support our patients. Stuart and Lieberman in their book, *The Fifteen Minute Hour*, write, "By being able to engage the person psychologically while laying on hands in the process of examining the body, the physician is in a unique position to help the patient correct whatever disturbance in homeostasis has precipitated the visit to the doctor." The total person needs the treatment of the mind, body and spirit for total healing.

Trust is an integral part of any good relationship, and because of this, those in the relationship allow themselves to become vulnerable to each other. Never is that more true than in the doctor-patient relationship when a patient's illness makes him dependent upon the healthcare provider and vulnerable to whatever treatment is required to improve his health. Some of the things that patients are asked to do in the course of their diagnosis and treatment are humiliating, degrading and painful. If a patient did not trust his physician to have his best interests in mind, then he would have a very difficult time undergoing all that might be required of him. Sir James Spence, a respected British physician, may have said it best: "The essential unit of medical practice is the occasion when, in the intimacy of the consulting room or sick room, a person who is ill or believes himself to be ill, seeks the advice of a doctor whom he <u>trusts.</u>"

As patients, our trust must extend beyond our doctors to include nurses and other healthcare providers, hospitals, health plans and the professions themselves. Over the past few years, I have had several major operations, thanks to years of competitive athletics and numerous sport-related injuries. If I hadn't trusted the anesthesiologist to put me to sleep safely, the nursing staff to monitor and care for me properly afterward or the physical therapists (who I swore were related to the Marquis de Sade) to rehabilitate me, then I could never have gone through all I did in order to get better. Recovery was frustrating, painful and lengthy for me at times but trust in my doctor and the various other health-care professionals kept me going and enabled my ultimate successful recovery.

Who among us really believes that the managed care organizations have our best interests at heart? It has been the lack of trust in managed care organizations, company health plans and the profession in general that has created the adversarial atmosphere that now permeates our society. Individuals within these organizations often do have our interests at heart, but the larger corporate structure is perceived as not worthy of our trust.

The main components of trust are competence, loyalty or advocacy of the other's best interest, honesty or truth telling and confidentiality. Failure in any of these areas can seriously erode trust. One can easily see how the doctor-patient relationship could be affected if a physician failed to meet the expectations of a patient in any of these areas. The perception on the part of most Americans is that managed care organizations fail the measures of trust when it comes to loyalty and truth telling.

In a survey conducted by Professor Mark Hall at Wake Forest University Medical School, the major factors associated with trust in a doctor are his communication skills and bedside manner. Doctors who appear confident in their decisions engender more trust than those who don't. Finally, the ability to choose a doctor based on knowledge and information rather than selecting from an unknown list of doctors is another strong predictor of trust. Because we'll all be patients one day, here are some questions patients and doctors alike can consider when evaluating their physicians (and maybe even ourselves):

A Question of Trust

1. Do you think your doctor will do whatever it takes to provide all the care you need?
2. Do you believe your doctor only thinks about what is best for you?
3. Are his or her medical skills current and what you expect?
4. Is your doctor both thorough and careful?
5. Does your doctor pay full attention to you when you are telling your story?
6. Does your doctor provide you with all your treatment options for your particular medical problem?
7. Do you trust your doctor's medical staff to tell you the truth and to look out after your best interests?
8. Are you willing to put your life in your doctor's hands? (Because you are.)

Difficult Doctors, Difficult Patients and Spirituality

"There is no such thing as 'the difficult patient.' Rather, there are specific difficult or challenging interactions for individual physicians—and not all physicians find the same interactions difficult."

–Frederic W. Platt, MD (Conversation Failure;
Case Studies in Doctor-Patient Communication)

"Damn, damn, damn," yelled the chief resident as he came out of the exam room. "I hate dealing with idiots who won't help themselves." Everyone, students and residents alike, looked at him in total surprise because the chief was known to be an easy-going, difficult-to-rattle kind of guy.

"What put a burr under your saddle, Denis?" one of the other third-year residents asked cautiously.

The chief laughed and took a big gulp from his bottled drink before replying. "Brendan, I just saw a sixty-year-old guy who's smoked two packs a day for forty years and who's coughing up crap from his lungs every day, and now is having a hard time breathing. He starts complaining to

223

me about all the doctors he's been to for his problem, that none of them have really helped him, and all every one of them does is tell him to stop smoking and take some useless medicines that never help. He 'knows' that smoking can't be doing this and that the other doctors just aren't smart enough to figure out the real problem. The damned guy's got COPD and emphysema that continues to worsen because he smokes like a damned chimney. What in the hell does he expect me to do and why is he wasting my damned time?"

The rest of the dozen students and residents gathered in the small doctor's dictating area just looked at each other and smiled ruefully. Most of the residents had experienced similar kinds of difficult patients before and knew that dealing with them was a fact of life in medicine. Many patients refused to take responsibility for their own lifestyle behaviors that had clearly produced adverse impacts on their health. What galled most physicians was that these same patients then had the audacity to expect their doctors to perform miracles. When the miracles didn't happen, they had the nerve to criticize the doctors trying to care for them. These were some of the most difficult patients to care for and to reach. It was frustrating and it had clearly gotten to Denis, the chief resident.

"Don't hide your true feelings so much, Denis," teased Brendan. "You need to get those feelings out. Don't keep them inside. Tell us how you really feel." At that, the whole room erupted in laughter. Brendan continued, "Hey, your guy's a piece of cake. Let me tell you about the winner I had earlier this week. This guy comes in complaining that he's been bringing up this thick green junk every time he coughs for the last four days. He also had a fever and upper respiratory symptoms. He wasn't a cigarette smoker but did enjoy a little of the 'evil weed' a few times a week. When I examined him he had a fiery red throat and some pus on his tonsils. I wrote him a few prescriptions, including an antibiotic for his obvious bronchitis and some nasal steroids to help open up his upper airways. I told him to drink plenty of fluids, stop smoking anything and get plenty of rest.

You know—the usual stuff. The next day, the guy calls me back and proceeds to give me holy hell because he wasn't feeling any better, and says he's going to complain to the chief of medicine about me."

Brendan was increasingly agitated as he recounted his story. His energy forced him to his feet and had him walking around the room as he continued with his story. "I tried to be calm and asked him what he'd done since he'd last seen me. First, he went snow skiing the afternoon after seeing me. Second, he didn't get his prescriptions filled until the morning of the day he called me. I know you all are going to find this hard to believe, but I was so shocked and surprised by his sheer stupidity and his lack of insight into his own behavior that I couldn't think of a thing to say."

Again, everyone broke into laughter. Brendan was of Irish ancestry and if anyone had the gift of the Blarney, he did. His father was a well-known radio personality with a gift for the gab and Brendan was an apple that definitely did not fall far from the tree. He liked to call himself "the old silver-tongued devil" and his wife, Geri, would often say that "If Brendan's bullshit were cement, he could pave his way around the world."

After the laughter stopped, Brendan resumed his story, "Seriously guys, I was dumbstruck. Then I could feel myself getting really pissed and that didn't help things in the least. I proceeded to ask him what he expected would happen with only one dose of a medicine. He then told me that he didn't like my tone of voice. I proceeded to tell him that I didn't like his attitude either and that only stupid people didn't know that when you had an illness for four days, it wasn't going to get better in one day, especially when you didn't take your medicine. Needless to say, things deteriorated from there. I got off the phone and knew that I hadn't handled things well."

Magen, one of the second-year female residents, jumped in at that point, "Brendan, it's great that you're sharing that story. We've all been there and have felt the same way you do when our patients acted that way. What did you do after you thought about your friendly little discussion?"

"First of all, Magen, I'm not sure I would have even shared that story with all of you if it hadn't been for Dr. Mary's Balint group. That really helped me to get in touch with my own feelings, or my own attitude, when dealing with difficult patients. I knew that I needed to call the jerk—er, ah—patient back and apologize even though it wasn't totally my fault. One thing I've learned from those groups is that we need to be somewhat above the fray. Remember what we were all taught in our group?"

All the residents shouted together with obvious glee, "The feeling is not the fact and the fantasy is not the act."

The Student turned to Magen with total confusion obvious on his face. "What's that all about?"

Magen was still laughing as she replied, "Dr. Mary Hall runs a Balint group for all the residents that, by the way, is also open to any interested student who might want to attend. Balint groups were begun in England to help doctors review their feelings when dealing with difficult patients or difficult situations that caused them emotional distress. What we're all laughing at is one of the phrases that have been repeated to us numerous times in the group. Dr. Mary has explained that just because we feel a certain way inside doesn't mean we have to make it a fact and keep that feeling with us. Likewise, just because we fantasize or think about doing something, we don't have to act on it. Brendan was upset but he didn't have to act on it even though it gives you a temporary feeling of relief."

The Student was impressed. Already in the brief period of time that he had dealt with patients, he'd experienced some real winners—or "wieners," as the other students liked to call them. He'd often wondered how many of the doctors had kept their cool when he had felt like jumping down the patient's throat. He liked the idea of being able to have a group discussion about some of the more difficult issues and thought that he just might participate in the future.

Brendan, the Student's resident for the day, called to him and told him to come see the next patient with him. It was a young man in his thirties who had been hit in the ribs while playing soccer. He complained that it hurt when he moved, when he coughed, or even when he took a deep breath. He'd never had any problems like this in the past and denied any difficulty with shortness of breath or coughing up blood. The chief resident then poked on the patient's ribs and listened to his lungs. "O.K., Student, what do you think I should do next?"

"I'd get a chest X-ray. No doubt about it," answered the Student.

"Why?" asked Brendan?

That question got the Student flustered. "Well, why not? Mr. Corcoran has a history of trauma to his ribs and he's obviously tender to touch. We've got to find out if he's got broken ribs. Isn't that right?"

"Yes, you're right about that, but the most important question to ask before you order ANY test is **'What will I do differently as a result of this test?'** If you're not going to do anything differently regardless of the results, then why order the test in the first place? Let me explain more in front of Mr. Corcoran because he obviously has a stake in this, and that's also a key element in practicing the Art of Medicine."

Oh God! Not another one of these residents talking about the Art of Medicine. My Advisor and some of his fellow believers in that Art stuff must have gotten to Brendan as well.

No, it'll take just a minute to cut the hook off.

The reason I am ordering the MRI is because I figure only a person with brain damage can hook their own nose.

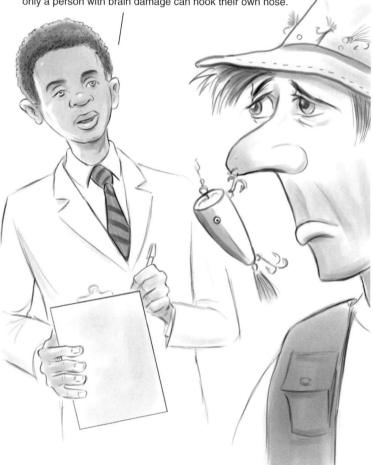

"As you saw, I examined Mr. Corcoran's ribs and he's awfully tender along the fourth rib on the right. He likely has a fractured rib based on his history and physical but he's having no difficulty breathing except with deep inspiration. That's good news because it means it's very unlikely that there's a punctured lung underneath. Even if the X-ray shows a fracture, we don't treat it any differently than if it was a severe contusion or bruise. Mr. Corcoran is going to be sore for about three weeks regardless of what we do. We're going to treat him with anti-inflammatories, ice the ribs down for forty-eight hours and keep him out of any athletics until one week after the pain is gone. So, why get the X-ray? You're not going to do anything different anyway."

The Student was really confused now. He'd never heard this kind of reasoning before. He had one burning objection to this concept. "What if you get sued because you didn't take the X-ray and you missed something?"

"Good thought, but this is where the Art of Medicine comes in. You always talk to the patient and explain your reasoning. Then you ask the patient what he would prefer you do. You then document it in his chart and make sure your patient knows to call you or return if he starts having any problems. Your job is to write down what those serious problems might be so the patient can refer to them later. Most people forget about forty percent of what they hear when physicians speak to them, so you'd better be sure to write down all the key points so that patients can take them home with them."

The chief resident turned to Mr. Corcoran. "Well you've heard all our discussion. What would you like us to do? Do you want some X-rays of your ribs or can you do without them?"

Mr. Corcoran got a big smile on his face. "Doc, that was a great explanation. Forget the X-ray. I don't need it and I can save some money for my insurance company and myself. If

I have problems, I'll come back and see you or see my personal physician. I really appreciate your honesty. If I don't need to get cooked by some X-rays, then let's not do it."

The Student and his resident wrote out his instructions, gave him the prescription and got him on his way. It was the last patient of the day and the Student had to run to make his mandatory lecture in the Art of Medicine series. This particular conference was going to be about the spiritual side of caring for patients. The Student got to the auditorium just in time to hear the introduction of the day's speaker, a Benedictine monk.

A Benedictine monk? A priest who lives in a monastery is speaking to our medical school class? What are they thinking? What could possibly be next? They're taking this Art of Medicine stuff way too far. Whoever designed this course has gone over the deep end. Scotty, please beam me back to the real world of medicine!

The speaker's opening remarks quickly brought the Student back to the classroom. "Good morning everyone. I'm Dr. Timothy Kelly. I'm here today to speak to you about Spirituality and Medicine. Hopefully, by the end of our time together, you'll come to understand, if not appreciate, the need for considering the spiritual aspect of your patients' lives. It's an integral part of most patients' lives and is extremely important to consider when your patient is faced with a serious or chronic illness, and especially at the end of life.

"I'm a licensed physician as well as a Benedictine monk. I know that's a very strange combination but I find that it's served me quite well in both of my ministries over the years. It may be surprising to many of you but the two professions have many things in common—but that's a whole different lecture. You may be surprised to learn that almost half of all US medical schools now have courses in Spirituality and Health. I normally am one of the teachers in Georgetown's one-semester course titled 'Religious Traditions and Health' that's required of all medical students there. Why are these courses becoming the norm? The answer may be surprising to you. It's because most patients want to be seen and treated as whole persons—that is persons with physical, emotional and spiritual dimensions. Ignoring any of these aspects of humanity leaves the patient feeling incomplete, and may even interfere with healing. Spirituality and religion are often used interchangeably and I will do so today, so please forgive me if it gets confusing.

"Many seriously ill patients use religious beliefs to cope with their illnesses, and there are many studies that support the wisdom of this position. These studies indicate the link between faith and health. Those with spiritual beliefs live longer, have fewer health problems, recover faster from surgery, have lower blood pressure and have much lower rates of depression and anxiety. Not bad, huh?"

Dr. Kelly proceeded to elaborate on all those points in a way that many in the auditorium had never heard before.

The Student was impressed. *If good health is your goal, then a spiritual belief seems to be a definite asset. I'd be so uncomfortable talking about this with any patient. Sure I go to church on Sundays once in a while, but who am I to speak to anyone about religion?*

"So, what should you as physicians do for your patients when it comes to spirituality? Simply put, physicians should acknowledge and respect the spiritual lives of their patients and keep any interventions patient-centered. What this means is taking a spiritual history much like you'd take a sexual history. Did you know that a consensus panel of the American College of Physicians suggested four simple questions that physicians might ask about this subject in their patients? They were:

1. Is religion or spirituality important to you in this illness?
2. Has faith been important to you at other times in your life?

① <u>Is</u> religion or spirituality important to you in this illness?

② Has faith been important to you at other times in your life?

③ Do you have someone to talk to about religious matters?

④ Would you like to explore religious matters with anyone?

3. Do you have someone to talk to about religious matters?
4. Would you like to explore religious matters with any-one?

"Just taking this spiritual history is often a powerful in-tervention in itself. Dr. Harold Koenig of Duke University may have said it best when he said, 'The physician can thus send an important message that he or she is concerned with the whole person, a message that enhances the patient-physician relationship and may increase the therapeutic im-pact of medical interventions.'

"I'll end my remarks to you today by saying that our call-ing as physicians is to cure sometimes, relieve often, but comfort always. If we have nothing else to offer, we can help our patients achieve an inner peace derived from their be-lief in a higher power. Thank you for listening."

Dr. Kelly finished and then proceeded to answer ques-tions from all those interested.

As the Student began to make his way out of the audito-rium, his Advisor approached him from behind. "What did you think? Do you buy into what Dr. Kelly was saying?"

The Student thought briefly before replying, "Yes, at some level I do. Some of my older family members who died and some of the nuns and priests who taught me in school had this great peace about them at the end. They also had a wonderful acceptance of serious illness that was be-yond me. I'm just not sure I know how to incorporate this into my practice in the future."

"Have you ever seen what you consider a miracle, Stu-dent?" asked the Advisor.

"No, sir. I haven't."

"Well, I have on several occasions. I call them miracles but others might call them medical events that are clearly be-yond my capacity to explain. I've been involved in caring for several patients who had extremely serious diseases that we were treating, albeit unsuccessfully, and somehow or another they seemed to resolve spontaneously. I have no explanation for it that makes any sense to me. All of these people had strong spiritual beliefs and I supported them in their belief system. It definitely wasn't our efforts that made them better, so I have to ascribe it to a higher power."

They continued their walk out of the auditorium and as they got ready to leave each other's company the Advisor had one final comment. "I know you think I'm crazy when I say these things to you but keep an open mind. As you treat more people, you'll see things that you won't be able to explain. Just be in awe of it and be grateful that you had the opportunity to be a part of it. See you next week."

The Student wasn't sure what to think. He knew there were many things he didn't understand but he hoped time would help him begin to sort through many of these things. It was all this soft science that got him the most confused.

✤ *Perspectives for Doctors* ✤

A group of nationally known experts in the field of medical interviewing and doctor-patient relationships conducted a survey in the early 1990s to assess the nature of physicians' frustrations with their practices and found that difficult, confrontational or challenging interactions accounted for up to 25% of an average primary care physician's practice. Imagine what that percentage might be today because of the changes brought about by managed care demands and increasing patient expectations. If a typical physician sees about 100,000 patients over a twenty-year career, then it might mean that he or she will have more than 20,000 troublesome visits or difficult patient encounters in a career. Isn't that something to look forward to?

That same survey indicated that physicians held the patients responsible for the frustrating visits 50% of the time.

They also noted communication skills and the nature of the practice setting as contributing factors, but rarely did doctors assume responsibility for their frustration. When marriages fail, rarely is a single party to blame because both parties often make some contribution to the ultimate demise of a marriage or, in this case, the doctor-patient relationship. If 15% of patients leave a practice yearly, as most surveys indicate (and most do so because of unhappiness with their doctor or their staff), that's a tremendous drain on the practice and requires constant recruitment of new patients.

There were seven major communication problems accounting for all this frustration:

1. Patients' lack or trust in or agreement with their physician
2. Patients presenting with too many problems
3. Patients' non-adherence with treatment plans
4. Patients' lack of understanding
5. Patients who are demanding or controlling
6. Patients with special medical problems (alcohol or drug abuse, psychiatric disorders, chronic pain)
7. Physicians' feelings of emotional distress secondary to patients

Female physicians participating in this survey were even more frustrated than their male colleagues about the number of patient problems, patient non-adherence to treatment plans and their own feelings of distress. Along with the inability to have a flexible schedule for personal family reasons, these are the major reasons why so many more women physicians choose to leave medical practice than do their male counterparts. Extreme frustration and no joy in our jobs are the biggest reasons why any of us choose to look elsewhere for employment.

At the Miles Institute for Health Care Communication, physicians were taught techniques for dealing with difficult doctor-patient interactions and how to minimize potential difficulties. Both doctors and patients can use these techniques, in the form of an easy-to-remember ABCDE acronym. Relationships are a two-way street so either party can take responsibility for noticing a problem and working to improve it.

Acknowledge—Either the doctor or the patient should acknowledge that there is a problem in the relationship and directly articulate the concern. Ask for help from the other person in solving the problem because relationships always involve two parties.

Boundaries—Both parties in any relationship need to know and understand their roles and responsibilities and the boundaries in that interaction. All of us need to have the rules or expectations clearly communicated to us. Patients need to ask what the boundaries are and physicians should inquire about patient expectations.

Compassion—An expression of caring or an act of compassion can make a huge difference in a difficult or emotional situation. Understanding the emotional state of the distressed party and letting him or her know that you are aware and empathize is imperative for the healing relationship.

Discover meaning—Try to understand the situation or the illness from the other's perspective. The doctor needs to understand how the particular illness is affecting the lifestyle of the patient or what it means to him, e.g., he saw his father get seriously ill in the same way. Patients need to try and understand what particular pressures might be impacting their doctors on a given day. As Stephen Covey advises in his *7 Habits* book, 'First, Understand the Other.' If we all do that, then many problems can be avoided.

Extend the system—Go beyond the conventional office relationship and use outside resources such as community agencies or support groups. No one practice can be all things to all people—and shouldn't be. Take advantage of the life experience and training of others to go beyond the obvious.

Spirituality is a very difficult concept to define, measure or evaluate. It may be the same as or different from religion for some. It has to do with whatever gives ultimate meaning and value to a person's life. Dr. Eric Cassell, a noted physician and ethicist, notes that when physicians attend to the body rather than to the person, they fail to diagnose suffering. When curing is no longer possible, there are still opportunities for healing. If time is taken to hear a patient's story at the end of life, then often the spiritual dimensions of suffering can be addressed. These can be simple tasks such as remembering others, deepening relationships, saying goodbye and forgiving.

Dr. Harold Koenig makes the point in his book, *The Healing Power of Faith*, that up to 90% of patients in certain parts of the country rely on religion for comfort and strength during times of serious illness. A recent review of over 1,200 studies of religion and health reported that at least two-thirds of the studies evaluated had shown significant associations between religious activity and better mental health, better physical health or diminished use of health services.

Anxiety, depression and loss of hope may complicate the course of many diseases and prevent patients from complying with recommended treatments, self-care activities or needed rehabilitation. Spirituality or religion can play a significant role in restoring emotional health back to many patients. Taking a spiritual history is still somewhat controversial but, by doing so, the physician signals to the patient that he or she cares about the patient's sources of hope and meaning during a serious illness. Think again about the great cardiologist Dr. Paul Dudley White's belief that to take care of the total person you had to consider the mind, the body and the spirit. Neglect one and you often will neglect a key part of that person's health.

Medications and Medical Errors

"There are several kinds of what is called noncompliance with taking prescribed medicines.

-There are those patients who do not take your prescribed drugs because they did not understand the instructions.

Learn to communicate in their language.

-There are those patients who do not take your recommended drugs because they do not trust your opinion.

Learn to build trust and respect.

-There are those patients who do not take your drugs because they make them feel bad.

Learn to hear these people. They are often correct."

–Dr. Clifton Meador
A Little Book of Doctor's Rules

Why they ever located the Pharmacy in the basement of the Medical Center was sure a mystery to the Student. It took forever to get here and it seemed so far away from the real action happening on the floors above. Spending time in the pharmacy was another one of those curriculum changes that had recently been instituted at the medical school and was now required of all medical students.

His first day on the rotation was spent at the local drug store with two other students observing the whole process of how prescription medications were obtained by patients. He had seen how medicines were brought and then stocked on the shelves. He had learned how physicians and their offices called in prescriptions for medicines. He had watched patients come to the counter and how they got totally confused by the whole process of insurance payments, co-pays and generic drugs and by the information about drugs that had to be provided to them. He'd also seen patients ask drug store personnel about over-the-counter medicines and realized that the store personnel often had little knowledge about many of the drugs.

Today was his first day in the actual hospital pharmacy and he didn't really know what to expect. He couldn't imagine it being very exciting. Just observing in the drug store yesterday was like watching paint dry—boring. He was so glad that he hadn't decided to go to pharmacy school instead of medical school, and that this rotation was only for two weeks. This particular rotation was going to be even worse since he'd be on it with a couple of his classmates he couldn't stand. They were the kings—and queens—of suck-ups. The only good thing about the pharmacy rotation was that he didn't have to take call, so at least he'd be home at a reasonable hour every day. He finally reached the pharmacy and slowly pushed open the door while looking for the Chief of Pharmacy, Magen O'Doyle.

"Hi, I'm Dr. O'Doyle. You must be our final medical student. Come on in here with the rest of the students. We're about to begin our orientation session. Would you like some coffee?"

"Uh, no thanks. Don't drink it," the Student mumbled as he found a seat and sat down.

He hated being the last one to get there. He felt like he was more noticeable to the teachers, especially since they were waiting for him.

What a bunch of brown-nosers! Had to be here early. Probably already asking questions.

Dr. O'Doyle's voice brought him back to reality. "Prior to coming on this rotation, most medical students have no idea of the magnitude of the problems associated with medicines in the United States. Let me spell out some facts for you. There were 300,000 hospital admissions this past year related in some way to adverse drug reactions. Three percent of the 33 million hospitalizations in 1997 had a preventable adverse event associated with them that cost an average of $2.7 million dollars per 700-bed teaching hospital. Nine out of ten patients don't take their prescription medicines properly. Fifteen percent of patients never get their prescriptions filled once they leave their doctors' offices. It's for these very reasons that every medical student is now required to spend time on this rotation. I say required because most students wouldn't venture down to the catacombs of the hospital unless forced to do so. I know that and that's fine with me. What I do hope is that you'll keep your minds open to what you'll be hearing over the next two weeks because the one thing that I can guarantee is that you will definitely see the adverse side effects of prescription medicines in your patients. It's inevitable but you can reduce your risk of serious problems if you pay attention to what you'll learn while you're here."

Dr. O'Doyle acknowledged the raised hand of one of the students, "Yes, Dr. DeKoskey."

"You can't be serious. One out of every five hospital admissions is related to problems associated with drug interactions or the side effects of drugs?"

"Serious as a heart attack. These problems occur predominately in older patients and for a variety of reasons. First, the metabolism of drugs in the body takes place primarily in the liver and the kidney. As we age, our metabolism slows so it takes less of a drug to exert the same effect. Therefore most of us should usually be taking lower doses of a drug, as we get older. Unfortunately, this often doesn't occur and that's where we encounter problems.

"Second, as we age, our bodies begin to wear down so we begin to have more and more medical problems requiring a number of different medicines to treat our various ailments. Let me give you a very practical example. Except for vitamins, most of you take no medicines on a regular basis. Your parents, on the other hand, take a number of medicines. The most common drugs that people take as they age are for cholesterol, blood pressure, arthritis, vitamin or herbal supplements and, in some women, hormones despite the adverse side effects noted in recent studies. Regardless of how safe they may seem, all medicines have side effects associated with them, and of course, they can produce drug-drug interactions.

"Third, the older we get, the more often we seem to get what we kindly call 'senior moments,' or what some of you call 'brain farts.' The hectic pace of our lives, our normal forgetfulness, and the complexity of taking many medicines at many different times during the day all contribute to problems with taking medications, whether too little or too much. Remember the statistic. Nine out of ten people do not take their medicines properly."

Dr. O'Doyle paused to see if she had everyone's attention. She did. "Who can tell me how many prescription medicines are available for use with patients today?"

"Five thousand," guessed one student.

"No, higher."

"Seventy-five hundred," ventured another student.

"No, I only wish there were that few, but there are over 17,000 prescription medicines on the market and available for patients today. And, according to the Pharmaceutical Research and Manufacturers of America (PhRMA), there were over 213,000 of what's classified as drugs available to people. How can we possibly remember all of them and how they might react with one another?"

Dr. O'Doyle paused again as she could still see the shocked looks on everyone's faces. "It's really a rhetorical question because the answer is that it's IMPOSSIBLE. None of us are that smart, but there are some things you can do to help yourself. For instance, these little pocket organizers or PDAs (personal digital assistants) like the Palm Pilot have programs that you can load onto them that provide information on drugs and their interactions. That one program alone would more than justify the cost of these hand-held devices many times over.

"Thanks in great part to managed care, there are more prescriptions than ever being written—over three billion in the year 2000. Nine out of ten prescriptions are now covered by some third-party payer. Direct-to-consumer advertising has also added to the cost of prescriptions. In 1995 pharmaceutical manufacturers spent $250 million on advertising to consumers and over $2 billion in 2000. You'd better know your medicines, or know where to find out the information about them, because there'll be more pressure on you than ever to write more prescriptions.

"Any questions? All right then, you've all got assignments, so let's get to it." The Student and two other classmates were to finish the morning in the pharmacy, reviewing drug orders, and then they were off to medical clinic in the afternoon. They, along with Dr. O'Doyle, began quickly sorting through the various physician orders to see if there were any incorrect medical orders or possible drug interactions.

Dr. O'Doyle quickly interrupted the group. "Here's a problem order we need to review. This particular doctor has ordered a couple of antibiotics as well as a cardiac medicine at a dose that is appropriate for a normal patient, but this patient has both kidney disease and liver disease. Does anyone want to explain why that's a potential problem? Devin?"

"Most drugs are primarily metabolized in the liver and excreted through the kidneys. If the liver doesn't metabolize properly or as expected, then the drug can build up in your system, causing toxicity. Likewise, if the kidneys aren't clearing waste normally, then more of a drug will stick around and there will be higher blood levels. With both liver and kidney disease, blood levels of a medicine can get dangerously high in a hurry and then you'll have the likelihood of all sorts of side effects. The classic example of this is the antibiotic gentamycin. When that gets too high, it can cause loss of hearing due to ototoxicity."

"Great job, Devin. So, what we need to do now is call the physician and discuss the issue with him so that we not only protect this patient, but also help educate the doctor for the future. Prior to a couple of years ago, we never checked orders like this but simply filled them. Thanks to the Institute of Medicine's report on medical errors in 1999, we've now focused our attention on some system errors in hospitals that could easily be corrected. This change in the way we do business has helped to reduce many potential adverse drug events, or ADEs."

The group continued to review orders for the next couple of hours and found three more potential problem orders. It gave them all a good feeling that they were having a direct impact on patient safety, plus it brought home the lessons of the morning in a very real way. When finally done, all the students headed to their various afternoon clinics. The Student had been assigned to the acute medical walk-in clinic. It usually meant lots of problems that were fairly simple. It was a great way to begin to see some of the kinds of problems that they'd see in private practice.

The Student's first patient was a young woman complaining of fever, runny nose, cough and mild sore throat. She said that she'd had the problem for the past two days and it was about the same. The Student then went to get his resident, Dr. Ava Mealia, who went to see the patient with him. After examining the young lady together, the resident sought out the attending, Dr. Lewis Sigmon, to review the case with her.

"Well, what do you think is the best course of treatment for your patient, Dr. Mealia?"

Dr. Mealia didn't hesitate a bit before answering, "I think this young lady has a little bronchitis so I'd like to put her on a Z-pack. That should take care of her problem nicely."

"Student, what do you think? Do you agree with Dr. Mealia?"

"Sure, seems like a reasonable approach to me."

Dr. Sigmon paused briefly before responding. "I agree with you that the patient has bronchitis but I can't agree with either the use of antibiotics, or the use of zithromycin if we did decide to use antibiotics. Let me explain my perspective on this. First, there is an increasing problem with antibiotic resistance today that is largely due to the overuse of antibiotics in non-appropriate situations, such as viral illnesses, as well as using antibiotics that are not targeted to the particular clinical situation.

"Most upper respiratory infections are viral illnesses and antibiotics just don't work on them. Most sore throats are also viral and antibiotics aren't needed then, either. I do understand that patients often ask for antibiotics because they either don't know better or they've been led to believe by past encounters with physicians that antibiotics are needed. Antibiotics do no one any good in these cases and increase the chances of resistance developing in bacteria. Already we have instances where we have a difficult time killing certain bacteria because of the problem of resistance. We shouldn't be adding to the problem. We all have to learn to be more responsible in our use of antibiotics.

"Second, if antibiotics were called for in this particular clinical situation, you need to think about using the most target-specific drugs possible. Let me put it into better perspective for you. If you were going to shoot a rat, you could use a .22-gauge rifle or a pistol. You wouldn't use an elephant gun. It's the same when you use antibiotics. If you treat a simple case of bronchitis with zithromycin, then you're using the elephant gun. Instead, we should use a target-specific drug, such as amoxicillin or a sulfa-trimethoprin combination. You reduce resistance and you save the big guns until a time when you really need them. Don't waste the big ammunition on the small game, or you won't have it for a serious infection. Make sense?"

The resident was obviously humbled and was honest in his reply. "Do you know that you're the first doctor who's explained it to me this way? Your analogy really helps me to understand it in a meaningful way. The whole problem of antibiotic resistance may have been explained to me in the past but I clearly missed it. Why don't more doctors say more about this and why doesn't our pharmacy do more to counsel physicians in this regard when they prescribe medicines?"

Dr. Sigmon gave a rueful smile. "Let me answer the second question first. Many physicians are threatened by anyone looking over their shoulders, even if it helps their patients in the long run. I have never personally understood that kind of thinking but many of the efforts to date to reduce antibiotic usage have met with resistance. It's generally easier to monitor antibiotic use in the hospital because the pharmacy has to fill the orders but most prescriptions are written in an outpatient setting, making it even more difficult to control their use. Fact of the matter is our ER doctors are some of our worst offenders when it comes to over-

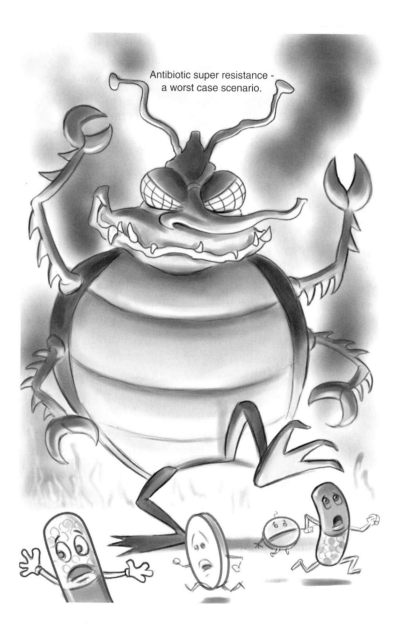

writing prescriptions. What they tell me is that they get a lot of pressure from patients to prescribe something because the patients feel so sick and that's why they've come to the ER. The doctors also say that they're so busy that they don't want to take the time to explain the reasons why antibiotics aren't really needed.

"The other reason that they write prescriptions for high-powered antibiotics is because they may not see the patients again, so they don't want to take a chance on missing some more exotic infection, and they give them a big gun. That thinking makes no sense to me but you should know that you'll hear it from some doctors at times. Patients can always come back in those rare instances where the bigger guns might be needed. Most of the time people feel better within forty-eight to seventy-two hours, regardless of what you do, so they don't return anyway. Here's a great fact sheet to give patients so they'll begin to understand the reasons behind your treatment. It will help cut down on problems in communication with your patients after they leave your office or the ER."

The resident and Student went back in to see their patient armed with these new facts and the patient information sheet. They finished up with that patient and quickly moved on to the next patient. It was a young woman complaining of urinary tract symptoms—urgency, frequency and some burning with urination. After the last patient, they were a bit reluctant to present the case because they were less sure of themselves. Once the resident had finished his presentation, Dr. Sigmon wanted to know what he'd recommend for treatment.

"I'd like to use some Cipro or Floxin for about seven days as I think that'll knock her UTI or cystitis right out."

Dr. Sigmon gave that little smile again and just shook his head. "Well, you're right about it knocking out whatever bug is causing your young lady's infection but I'm going to have to pound on you again. We've seen a great deal of resistance develop in recent years to traditional antibiotics used in uncomplicated UTIs but it doesn't mean they shouldn't be used. Do either of you know the resistance rate to various antibiotics here at this hospital?"

Both the Student and the resident shook their heads in the negative.

Dr. Sigmon pulled a slip of paper from her pocket. "Each month the hospital publishes the rates of antibiotic resistance for various medications for specific illnesses. For instance, under urinary tract infections, it shows that 10% of UTIs are resistant to the combination of trimethoprim-sulfamethoxasole while your Cipro has a 5% resistance rate. Since this is an uncomplicated case, I would still suggest using the least broad antibiotic possible because the odds are in your favor. The medicines you're suggesting using are too broad and should be saved for the more complicated cases. Again, the other problem with the broader spectrum meds is the increased risk of developing resistance. So, let's cool it with the big guns and use the three-day course of the Septra or Bactrim. O.K.?"

The resident nodded in agreement. He felt like a chastised schoolboy but knew that Dr. Sigmon was suggesting the course of action that was best for the patient. On the other hand, Dr. Sigmon walked away thinking that it would take a good deal of positive reinforcement but things could be changed for the better, and it had to start with the younger doctors and students.

❖ *Perspectives for Doctors* ❖

In 1999 the Institute of Medicine (IOM) issued a report titled "To Err is Human." The central point in that report was indisputable—too many patients are suffering severe consequences that could, and should, be avoided. The IOM estimated that between 44,000 and 98,000 patients die each year as a result of preventable mistakes made in hospitals. These mistakes include medication mix-ups, faulty diagnoses, wrong surgeries and hospital-acquired infections because doctors and hospital staff didn't do something as simple as washing their hands. Total national costs (lost income, lost household production, disability and healthcare costs) of preventable adverse events (medical errors resulting in injury of some kind) are estimated to be between $17 and $29 billion, of which healthcare costs represent over one-half.

The shocking part of all these numbers is that the IOM report likely **under**estimates the extent of preventable medical injuries for a few important reasons. First, they are solely based on data extracted from medical records and most injuries and most errors are not recorded in the medical record. Second, the IOM estimates are low because they don't include outpatient injuries or errors. There is no reason to believe that the percentage of errors should be any less in this setting. Finally, in-depth studies reveal even higher rates of problems than in the IOM report. Dubois reported that 20% of deaths from heart attacks, pneumonia and strokes were preventable. Bedell reported that 64% of in-hospital cardiac arrests were preventable. Got your attention yet?

I may have gotten your attention but the previous report has not gotten the attention of those charged with educating medical students and residents on the subject. A recent research letter in the *Journal of the American Medical Association* (*JAMA*, Sept. 2001) reported that only 16% of all internal medicine clerkships in the survey had formal lectures on adverse drug reactions/interactions. Sadly, 35% of clerkship directors had little or no familiarity with the IOM's report on medical errors and how to reduce them.

So what can and is being done to reduce medical errors? And why don't we hear more about the problem? It's hard to believe but there hasn't been a champion who's come forward to move the healthcare system into action to make the needed changes. Surprisingly, consumers are silent on this issue. The media only report anecdotal cases of problems. Hospital accrediting and licensing organizations only touch on the problem of medical errors peripherally when performing their inspections, and even these minimal efforts are met with resistance due to the increased costs associated with fixing the problem. Providers are leery of systematically uncovering and learning from errors because of the fear of being hauled into court.

Another factor contributing to medical errors, and especially adverse drug events, is the lack of complete information on a patient. When patients see multiple providers in different settings, none of whom have all the medical information about that patient, it's easy to see how something can go wrong. While in the ER, I used to see patients who didn't know what medicines they were taking, what their actual diagnoses were and what their test results really showed. I felt like a pilot flying blind. In most cases I had no way to get their medical records so I had to guess at the best course of treatment or the best drugs to give them. Without that information, I could have given a medication that interacted with a drug they were already taking and caused even further problems.

Finally, two of the biggest obstacles to needed reform are employers and group purchasers of health insurance. Very few are truly concerned about quality of care or safety but are only focused on one thing—cost. Likewise, most, if not all, third-party payment systems provide little incentive for a healthcare organization to improve safety, nor do they recognize or reward safety or quality.

So, what's the answer? Consumer groups with huge clout, such as the American Association of Retired Persons (AARP) and professional physician organizations, need to put safety and quality of care issues as priorities on their agendas. There is no excuse for our system of healthcare to have so many preventable deaths.

The problem of medical error is not fundamentally due to lack of medical knowledge. Simple measures of known effectiveness, such as unit dosing, marking the correct side before surgery and twenty-four-hour availability of pharmacists and emergency physicians, are often ignored. Healthcare refuses to learn what other industries such as airlines have already learned: Safe performance cannot be expected from workers who are sleep deprived, who work double or triple shifts or whose job designs involve multiple or competing urgent priorities.

Since their introduction in the 1940s, antibiotics have been the primary treatment for bacterial infections and have often been called "miracle drugs." One of the major problems facing medicine today is the emergence of drug-resistant microorganisms or bacteria, thanks to the inappropriate overuse of antibiotics. National medical organizations, including the Infectious Disease Society of America (IDSA), have identified antibiotic resistance as a major concern. This resistance was originally confined to hospitals but is now emerging as a community problem. Why is this happening and what can be done about it?

It's clear that antibiotic resistance is directly proportional to the volume of antibiotic consumption. The fewer antibiotics used, the less resistance develops. Studies have indicated that 20% to 50% of antibiotic prescriptions in community settings are believed to be unnecessary. The reasons attributed to this unnecessary use of antibiotics are unreasonable patient expectations or demands (wanting antibiotics when they are not indicated, as in viral infections), inadequate time to explain to patients (or parents) why antibiotics are unnecessary, misdiagnosis of nonbacterial infections and the desire to keep good patient relationships even though antibiotics may not be efficacious. Other concerns include fear of litigation, cost-saving pressures to substitute therapy for diagnostic tests, misleading advertising by drug companies and productivity incentives in managed care organizations. Even the use of antibiotics in animals to promote growth and treat infections may be a contributing factor in people because as resistance develops in animals, it may also be passed to the human population.

What can be done to slow the increasing rate of resistance? The answer requires action on the part of both physicians and patients. Physicians should not accommodate patient requests for unneeded antibiotics, should use targeted antibiotics rather than broad-spectrum medicines, should educate patients about the proper use of antibiotics and should not prescribe antibiotics for viral illnesses. Patients should ask their doctors to prescribe the most directed antibiotic with the most appropriate spectrum of activity for their problem and not to prescribe antibiotics for viral illnesses.

Sore throats are the second-most common symptomatic reason for seeking medical care in the United States. Most sore throats are due to upper respiratory tract viruses. The only cause of sore throat warranting treatment is beta-strep infection and it is cultured in children between 15% and 36% and in adults between 5% and 17%. Why then are 76% of adults diagnosed with sore throat treated with antibiotics? And when they are treated, why are they treated with the wrong antibiotic? A recent survey in *JAMA* (Sept., 2001) found that non-recommended antibiotics were used in the treatment of sore throats 68% of the time. Instead of using penicillin or erythromycin (for penicillin-allergic patients), patients were given extended-spectrum macrolides or fluoroquinolone antibiotics. Not only is this practice much more costly, but it greatly increases the likelihood of resistance.

Drug interactions are obviously an extremely serious problem with tremendous impact on the health and finances of this country, not to mention on the people who have these reactions. Some of the symptoms of drug interactions include confusion, falling, weight loss, dizziness and changes in behavior or moods.

I can't tell you how many times I would ask patients in the ER what medicines they were currently taking so that I could safely write what was needed that night, or to see if their current meds could be causing some of the symptoms they were having. Most of the time, patients did not know exactly what they were taking or in what dosage. I heard time and time again, "I'm not exactly sure what I'm taking but I think it's for high blood pressure and it's a little blue pill." Whoopdeedo! That kind of information didn't help me a bit.

Reducing medical errors is a problem for all of us to address. We can't be passive but have to be actively engaged in the entire process, especially when it comes to the care and treatment of patients. An informed, engaged patient is the best help for all of us. Get involved locally with your healthcare institution and work toward implementing systems to reduce medical errors and adverse events.

Managed Care, Technology and Other Potential Barriers to the Art of Medicine

---

There were three medical specialists standing at the gates of heaven. St. Peter said to the first, "And what have you done to be able to enter heaven?"

"I'm a breast surgeon and have helped numerous women."

"Enter, you've done a wonderful job."

To the second he said, "And what about you?"

"I'm an oncologist and have taken care of those dying from cancer."

"Enter, you really helped many while on earth."

To the third he said, "Yes, and you?"

"I was a director of an HMO."

"Enter, but you'll have to leave after three days."

Most of the medical school faculty was seated in the auditorium listening to the Dean of the Medical School introduce one of the speakers for the morning presentation. Scattered throughout the audience were a number of residents as well as some students. The medical director for the state's largest HMO and their marketing director would be discussing managed care with the faculty. The medical staff was there to hear the details of a proposed new arrangement for payment of clinical services to the medical school faculty for care rendered at the hospital. Before the visit, many of the faculty openly shared their disgust with the managed care organization. Reimbursement was currently at around sixty-five cents for every dollar billed, but the HMO was proposing lowering that to fifty cents on the dollar.

Academic medical schools had been especially hard-hit financially by the new managed care environment. These organizations didn't care that one of the biggest roles of medical schools like this one was the education of many different kinds of health professionals, from doctors and nurses to physical therapists and respiratory care specialists. They only wanted to reimburse for the patient care component and not for any part of the education of future physicians. This didn't begin to cover the costs of many services provided in the academic centers, so most were dependent on state funding and private donors to keep their institutions afloat financially. Fund-raising was a constant chore. It was often the large donations that enabled the academic centers to attract and retain the best faculty because without these donations, they couldn't compete with the pay that doctors could make in private practice.

The managed care presentation began on time. It was extremely slick and well organized using the latest in audiovisual technology to illustrate the points in the presentation. The bottom line: The HMO wanted to lower all fees, just as most everyone had expected. There was no applause when the presentation was finished and the anger in the room was almost palpable. The floor was quickly opened to questions.

One of the Ob-Gyn surgeons stood up first and asked, "Do my colleagues and I get reimbursed differently if we have an excellent record of getting patients home sooner or use surgical techniques that reduce the recovery time for our patients? For example, if I do a hysterectomy vaginally versus abdominally, the patient generally goes home sooner and has a lot fewer problems after surgery."

"No, we reimburse at the same level."

"So, if we just use your reimbursement scheme as a guide, what you're saying is that quality of care and length of stay don't matter. Better care doesn't improve the reimbursement."

"No, that's not what we're saying. We've just decided to reimburse by procedure and not use other factors. I know on the surface it may not sound right but it works out the same at the end."

The surgeon made one final angry comment before sitting down. "It may not make a difference to you but it makes a big damned difference to the patient. I guaran-damn-tee you that if it was your wife having it done, she'd want the surgeon who could do the vaginal approach and who would get her home sooner with fewer problems and a faster recovery time." The audience burst into applause as he sat.

Next, a general medicine faculty member raised another issue. "I primarily see patients in a clinic setting. I try to keep down the number of X-ray or lab tests that I do by spending time with the patient and making a proper diagnosis. Do I get compensated differently for this when compared to other physicians who may order many more tests and still come to the same conclusion?"

"No, we don't currently break our data down this way to differentiate."

"Don't you think you should? What incentive is it for the physician to spend more time with the patient? The more patients he can see, the more he can bill. Lab tests of various kinds cost a lot more than physician time."

"It's something that we will likely look into for the future."

Angrily, the physician replied, "It makes no sense. You talk about your concern about quality of care and avoiding

Nah, I don't think we need any lab tests.
These things have a way of working themselves out.

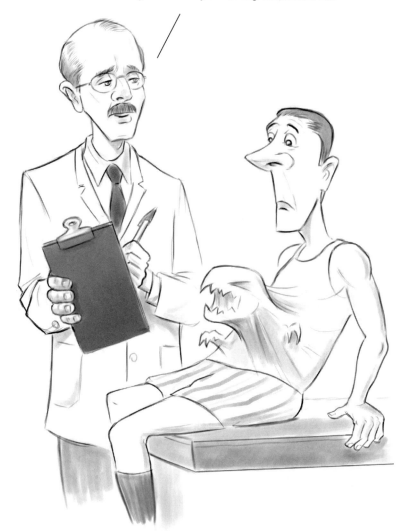

unnecessary testing, yet you don't do simple profiling that would help with this. You've had all the data for years but you just don't want to go to all the trouble of analyzing it and using it. It's easier for you just to cut our fees across the board."

One of the more popular pediatricians then stood up to speak. "We in pediatrics and many of the physicians in practice don't have any procedures or fancy tests that we do on our patients. We simply talk to them or their parents, examine them, and maybe do some simple testing. We may spend a half-hour or more with a single patient trying to make a diagnosis or do some counseling. Yet, one of my colleagues in cardiology can do a stress test or my GI medical friends can perform an EGD (esophago-gastric duodenoscopy) in the same amount of time and they are reimbursed at considerably higher rates, yet the time spent with the patient is the same. Is this fair?"

"What you're referring to was the system of compensation set up long ago. It goes back to the early '30s when Blue Cross and Blue Shield first began. We are simply following the common practice in the industry. Procedures do get higher reimbursement. It's just the way the system is."

Losing all semblance of civility because of the unfairness of it all, the pediatrician sharply answered, "Sir, don't piss on me and then try and tell me that it's raining. There are many other things you've changed in the past that were common practice in the industry when they were good for your HMO financially. I'm sure you could change this if you chose to but it's not in your best interest—only our patients'." Again, the entire audience broke into appreciative applause.

The next physician to go to the microphone was one of the oncology specialists. "We are an academic institution dedicated to teaching and research. We are at the leading edge of the battle with cancer. Some of what we do is clinical trials to see if new treatments are better than what is currently available. It's the only way to break new ground and make advances in the treatment of cancer. We already know that HMOs don't reimburse for teaching time despite the fact that it leads to better medical care for the future. Now you don't want to provide any compensation for clinical practices that may advance medicine because you say some of what we do is 'experimental.' How do you respond to this?"

The medical director chose to answer that question, "Well, it's not our job to do research, but to provide proven medical care to the patients in our HMO. We don't want to take the liability of paying for something that's untried and may increase our risk. We also believe it's not our job to fund research, but it is the duty of state and federal government as well as private contributors to fund needed research."

The questioning continued with the general tenor of most remaining the same. It was clear that the physicians wanted some way to differentiate providers based on the quality of care provided and the time spent with the patient. This HMO and most others were strictly concerned with the financial bottom line. The quality of care provided came in a distant second as far as the attention paid to it in terms of physician profiling. The meeting finished with neither side giving ground on the points it tried to make. It was always a fine balance between wanting to care for patients and paying what was a fair wage. Because the HMO had so many patients enrolled under its plan, the fear on the part of the faculty was that the loss of so much business would mean fewer patients from whom the residents and students could learn. The final decision about whether or not to continue with the HMO plan would be made by the medical center faculty group, but it would not be without considerable debate and a great deal of controversy. For the residents and students, it was a good glimpse into the debate occurring in medical practices all across the United States.

The Student left the auditorium and quickly hurried to cardiology rounds. The attending this week was Dr. Marion Limacher. She was one of the leaders of a huge nationwide study evaluating heart disease in women. Until the 1990s, all of the major studies evaluating heart disease were conducted on men and the data simply extrapolated to women. It took years to realize that this wasn't good medicine, since women often presented with very different symptoms than men when they had cardiac disease. Until some of the more recent research, it was thought that women didn't have to worry about heart attacks as long as they were menstruating since their estrogen seemed to have a protective effect on the heart. It was a real surprise to find that many younger women had heart disease as well.

Dr. Jape Taylor was also rounding on cardiology that morning with Dr. Limacher. The Student became extremely nervous because Dr. Taylor was somewhat of the "old" school. He was often made fun of by some of the residents because of his belief that examining the patient would often lead to the correct diagnosis faster and more cheaply than all the technological tests available today. He hated the reliance on technology alone and would often say sarcastically to some of the residents, "The motto of you younger guys seems to be 'If all else fails, see the patient.'"

The senior resident, Dr. Ray Bianchi, presented the first patient seen that morning on rounds to the group. "Mrs. Benson is a sixty-five-year-old white female who presented to her primary care physician with a three-month history of burning in the epigastric area. She had been treated with various GI medicines including histamine blockers and Prilosec without relief. She had a history of borderline hypertension and mild elevated cholesterol. She came to the ER two nights ago complaining of epigastric pain and jaw

261

pain associated with some mild shortness of breath when walking. The ER doctor was astute enough to realize that women often have atypical pain symptoms associated with cardiac disease. He did an ECG that showed marked is-chemic changes. She was admitted that night and had a car-diac stress test the next morning. It was markedly abnormal after exercising for only a few minutes. Later that day Mrs. Benson had a cardiac cath and two-vessel angioplasty with stents. She denies any epigastric pain since the angioplasty even though she's off of all GI medicines."

Dr. Limacher took over then. "Anyone care to tell me the most important lesson that we should all remember from this patient?"

One of the other residents raised her hand. "It sounds like the epigastric pain wasn't truly stomach pain but was really referred cardiac pain. According to some of the recent data, women often have unusual symptoms of coronary artery disease. I think the lesson we all need to remember is that we need to be very suspicious when women present with pain, especially when they have numerous cardiac risk fac-tors like Mrs. Benson had."

"Great answer. Women generally develop coronary dis-ease later in life thanks to the protective effect of estrogen. It was hoped that starting women on hormone replacement therapy might further delay the risk of cardiovascular disease as well as treat some of the other problems of menopause such as osteoporosis, hot flashes and vaginal dryness. Unfortunately, the risk of cancer seems to be in-creased and it does little for heart disease. The real key for women is to educate them on the need to pay attention to their own risk factors for heart disease and take appropriate action after consultation with their doctor."

The next patient was presented to Dr. Taylor by one of the junior residents. "Mr. Atwell is a twenty-three-year-old man who was sent to our clinic by his primary care physician for evaluation of a cardiac murmur that was picked up on a routine physical. He just got back here a few minutes ago after having the diagnostic tests done that I'd ordered when he first came to the clinic a few hours ago. I reviewed his chart when he first came in and thought I'd save him some time by ordering an ultrasound, echocardiogram and stress test prior to our seeing him. Unfortunately, they were only able to do the first two tests today. I thought maybe we could all see the patient together after we reviewed the tests."

Dr. Taylor's face had gotten redder and redder the longer the presentation continued. He finally had enough and interrupted the resident. "Are you telling me that you ordered all those tests without even seeing the patient?"

The resident smiled and nodded his head affirmatively. "Yes, sir," he said with obvious pride.

Dr. Taylor's mouth gaped open and he just stared at the resident in amazement. "I can't believe it. Where have you been for the last few years? What have we been trying to teach you on this service? I know you think I'm an old fart who needs to get with it and begin using more of today's wonderful technology with patients, but this is ridiculous. It's no wonder that healthcare costs have gone through the roof and people are looking to managed care to help control them. What were you thinking? How can you possibly order a test without talking to the patient to get a history and examining him? It's about taking care of people and listening to their story. It's not just about making a diagnosis. I can't believe this, especially in a twenty-three-year-old man," he added angrily.

The resident was taken aback by the outburst but was smart enough not to say much. He'd learned that when you find yourself in a hole, the best thing you can do is to stop digging.

Dr. Taylor was still livid. "I know that in some private practices as well as some of the other medical services in this hospital, ordering tests prior to seeing the patient is almost routine practice. The GI guys are famous for this. They order CT scans of the abdomen for patients who are referred to them or schedule endoscopies for epigastric pain without trying a course of medicine to see if this solves or helps the problem. You can learn so much from talking to patients. You may eventually need testing but it can be focused and, in this way, you save time, money and the possible complications that accompany any test. I don't believe that this practice is good medicine. Eventually, you all will have to decide the best way to practice medicine for yourself. All that I ask you to do is please think about how you'd want one of your loved ones treated, and then apply that same yardstick to how you treat every patient." Dr. Taylor then turned to Dr. Limacher. "Do you agree with what I've said, Marion?"

Dr. Limacher had a serious look on her face as she replied, "You bet I do, Jape. This is not the way we want to practice medicine, nor the way we think people should be treated. I can see how it might save some time for the patient but it increases costs tremendously and it uses technology in the wrong way. Technology is not a screening tool but should confirm your tentative diagnosis or help point the physician toward a specific therapy. Anyone have anything to say before we go see the patient?"

No one did so the entire group went to examine the patient. Dr. Taylor introduced the group to Mr. Atwell and then proceeded to ask a number of questions as part of the history taking process. When done, he asked one of the first-year residents to show everyone how to conduct the actual hands-on examination. "Dr. Fox, I know that you'd like to become a thoracic surgeon one day so it might behoove you to learn how to conduct a physical examination." Dr. Fox quickly moved to examine the patient by pulling out his stethoscope and placing it on the patient's chest in various places. When done, he turned and put his stethoscope away.

Dr. Taylor just stared at Fox, shook his head in wonderment and said, "Are you done?"

"Yes, sir. I think I've made the diagnosis and believe we can help Mr. Atwell with a little surgery."

"Unbelievable, Dr. Fox. One thing I like about you: You may be wrong, but you're never in doubt. I'm glad you're considering surgery because a cardiologist you'll never make. When you perform a physical examination on the heart and lungs, there are a number of things that should be done if you want to do it correctly. First of all, we inspect the chest without clothes. We then put our hands on the chest and palpate to determine thrills or other abnormal signs. Finally, we auscultate or listen to the heart and lungs, but we place the patient in different positions to diagnose various problems." Dr. Taylor proceeded to demonstrate to the group what he meant by each step of the process.

"Before we look at the ultrasound or echocardiogram, does anyone want to hazard a guess as to Mr. Atwell's diagnosis after hearing the answers to the questions I posed and knowing what we found on the physical exam?" Dr. Taylor asked.

At first, no one uttered a sound and all appeared to be looking anywhere but at Dr. Taylor. Everyone was afraid of incurring any more of his wrath that day. Finally, one of the medical residents, Dr. Ray Bianchi, raised his hand. "Yes, Dr. Bianchi, you wish to hazard a guess?"

"Dr. Taylor, I believe this man has a benign cardiac murmur often called a functional murmur. He's in excellent shape. He has none of the physical attributes of Marfan's and denies taking steroids to build muscle mass. I've played a fair amount of sports in my time and I saw that in a few other well-conditioned athletes, both men and women."

Dr. Taylor beamed approvingly. "Nice job, Dr. Bianchi. It took guts to go out on the limb and expose your thinking like that, especially when I've been so tough on your colleagues today. I concur with your diagnosis. Let's review the technology to see if it agrees with what we think."

The tests proved to be completely normal which, by this time, was no big surprise. The lesson to the group was brought home in dramatic fashion. No tests were really needed but if the patient or some other group needed a confirmation, then just one of the tests would have been more than sufficient for that purpose. Dr. Limacher nicely reinforced all these points with the group before sending them off to lunch.

✢ *Perspectives for Doctors* ✢

There is no doubt that managed care organizations (MCOs) such as health maintenance organizations (HMOs), individual practice organizations (IPOs) and preferred provider organizations (PPOs) have had a positive impact on lowering healthcare costs. They have definitely "trimmed the fat off the meat" of the healthcare bone, to use an old analogy. Before their rise to popularity in the mid to late 1980s, there was little competition in medicine and healthcare costs went largely unchecked. Employers were seeing increases in healthcare costs of 20% annually. These skyrocketing medical benefit costs were often blamed for the inability of certain companies to compete. It was estimated in the 1980s that medical benefits alone added $700 to the cost of every new car. Employers began to scream for something to be done and MCOs in many different shapes and sizes arose to try and fill that need.

Today, MCOs generally work in the following way. They contract with a healthcare provider to render services for a specific fee—whether the provider is a hospital, physician or other provider, such as a nurse practitioner, physical

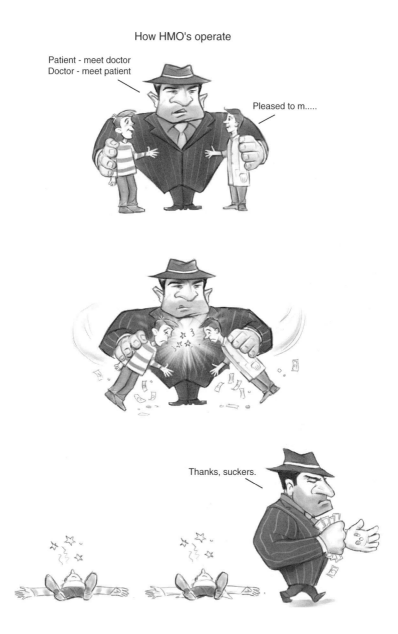

therapist or someone else providing a service to the patient. The MCO then bundles this into a specific premium or cost and sells this package to an employer for a set fee. The employer then defines a benefit package for its employee group, based on what it is willing to pay.

If the employer wants to offer an HMO to its employees, it provides a fixed amount of money to the employee per month and the employee then selects an HMO to provide all services to the employee. The employer does nothing further and has less to do than with conventional medical plans. Employers have almost forced many employees to join tightly managed insurance plans and have held down premiums as a result.

Aggressive purchasing practices among employers abound and include competitive bidding, RFPs (requests for proposals) and one-year contracts. These are hardball tactics and not partnerships, and companies seem to care only about the bottom line—so that's what insurers and MCOs try to deliver.

Employers may talk about quality but they often mean customer service. A Robert Wood Johnson Foundation survey indicated that 60% of employers had contractual requirements for provider access but barely one-third demanded annual improvements in clinical quality. General Motors is one of a handful of companies that rewards employees by reducing premiums if employees choose a health plan with high levels of quality care and preventive medicine. Employers can talk quality but until they change their contracts to reward quality and not just low cost, things won't change. Like any pendulum that swings, the MCO pendulum has now swung too far in the other direction with cost pressures being constantly applied to physicians, hospitals and other healthcare providers.

Managed care is a concern in that it has impacted the teaching of basic skills in medical school. Several studies in recent years note the declining medical examination skills of medical school graduates. It has become such a concern that the National Board of Medical Examiners is considering testing for clinical skills in the future. A recent study by physicians in two New York City hospitals demonstrated that International Medical Graduates (IMGs) performed significantly better than US medical school graduates on thirteen skills associated with abdominal examinations. These were not poor students but had graduated in the top quarter of their classes and were from sixty-three different medical schools.

One possible explanation for the decline in medical skills is that the access to patients for clinical teaching has decreased. This is another example of how managed care has had a negative impact on clinical medicine. One-third of total medical school revenues come from the clinical care provided by clinical faculty members of medical schools, so they are very vulnerable to third-party reimbursement. These MCOs, along with Medicare regulation, limit the ability of medical students to take histories or perform supervised physical examinations or procedures. The managed care competition has also been the reason for the merger, acquisition or closure of many hospitals, and thus further limited the number of patients available for clinical teaching as well.

Technology has brought many wonderful diagnostic advances to medicine but, like many other advances, it has to be used properly to obtain the greatest good. When I first started doing emergency medicine in 1976 in a small rural North Carolina community, I had no CT scans or ultrasound capability available in the hospital so I had to ship patients almost thirty miles away. When head trauma, abdominal trauma, or a possible ectopic pregnancy came to the ER, I had to rely on my physical exam skills and not technology to help me make the correct diagnosis. It was very scary, but I venture to say that my examination skills are far better than many of today's graduates because I couldn't rely on technology to do the diagnosing for me. In some ways, technology has made physicians lazy and less skillful. In reality, technology should be used to help confirm or deny your initial diagnosis.

Dr. J. Willis Hurst, former professor and chair of cardiology at Emory University, stated in an article for Medscape in 2001 "the major cause for the deterioration of clinical skills is the failure of attending physicians who teach to spend time with medical residents discussing the physiologic basis for heart sounds that they hear." He also lays blame at the ready availability to physicians of high-tech procedures, such as echocardiography and cardiac catheterization in the absence of any challenge of themselves or their trainees to auscultate before the exam or of making predictions about what the findings will be. He strongly believes that it is the attending physician who is at fault if a resident leaves a training program without the ability to examine a patient. I believe that says it all and throws down a real challenge to today's teachers.

What Every Doctor and Patient Need to Know—Real Wellness

Even at 6:45 in the morning, the Coronary Care Unit (CCU) was teeming with activity. The night-shift nurses were giving reports to the day-shift nurses who were just coming on duty to begin a long twelve-hour shift. The medicine team had already begun rounding on their patients. The three residents on the team who had been on call the night before were telling the rest of the group about the admissions for that night.

Two of the new admissions were men and the other was a woman. All were overweight and had done little or no exercise in recent years despite all the public health efforts encouraging exercise as a way of reducing the risk of heart attacks. All three of the patients were smokers, so not only were their hearts at greater risk, but their lungs were likely to be damaged as well. The last admission was just being presented to the group by one of the second-year residents when the Student arrived at the CCU.

"Mr. Cornelius is a fifty-eight-year-old gentleman who came to the ER this morning suffering from chest pain of several hours' duration. He also complained of shortness of breath, pain in his jaw and neck and feeling like an elephant was sitting on his chest. He's a one-pack-a-day cigarette smoker, has diabetes that he takes a pill for—he wasn't sure what—takes a blood pressure medicine and exercises rarely. He has no family history of heart disease, and both his parents died of cancer. We stabilized him in the ER, got him to the CCU, but did not begin antithrombolytic agents because he'd waited too long before coming to the ER. He's done well except for some isolated short runs of ventricular tachycardia."

The group was still fairly sleepy so there were no additional comments as they went into Mr. Cornelius's room. "Good morning, sir. We're this month's medical team and we'll be taking care of you while you're in the hospital. We wanted to come visit and see how you're doing today. How are you feeling this morning as compared to last night?"

"One hell of a lot better. I thought someone was sitting on my chest last night and I just couldn't catch my breath. You guys saved my life," the patient grunted sleepily.

"Mr. Cornelius, I hate to say it, but you didn't do much to help the situation. Why did you wait so long to come to the hospital?"

"Well . . . at first, I figured it might go away, that it might just be gas or some other stomach problem. As it got later and later, I didn't want to wake my wife. Thought maybe I could hold out until the morning and see my own doctor. Finally, I got so scared that I called the rescue squad."

"Didn't you recognize any of the warning signs of heart attack?" one of the other residents asked. "Even our medical students knew what was wrong with you, with all the symptoms you had." All the residents laughed at that last remark but none of the medical students found it especially funny.

"No, didn't give it much thought. I did, however, vow never to touch another cigarette, if I made it through this heart attack."

"Good, Mr. Cornelius. Stick with that resolution. It will definitely help you to live longer. Judging from your blood work and the cardiac monitoring we did during the night, it looks like you're doing a bit better. This is just a quick run-through to introduce you to everyone. Some of us will be back to see you later to spend a bit more time doing a little patient education with you. O.K., ladies and gentleman, time to write some orders and head for Grand Rounds."

It was another Grand Rounds presentation and the title of today's lecture was "A Different Paradigm for Preventive Medicine in the New Millennium." The students and residents had no idea what to expect but the general betting was that it would be boring beyond belief. The only thing that they couldn't figure was why it was going to take two people to team-teach the presentation.

One of the third-year medical residents, Dr. Dan Davis, could be heard commenting to a group of other residents as they walked down the hall, "I don't understand why all the faculty are making such a big deal about getting to this lecture. What could possibly be new about preventive medicine? Isn't it fairly simple? You find out what each patient's risk factors are, and then you try to get him to do something about them. Duh! It doesn't take rocket science." The group's laughter was suddenly cut short when they heard a voice behind them speak.

Dr. David Citron was one of the older, most respected faculty members who had been in private practice for many years before moving to the teaching faculty. His experience, coupled with his ability to connect with patients, made him revered among the residents and students.

"Dr. Davis, I couldn't help overhearing your learned insights into today's presentation. All that I can suggest to you is that based on many years of experience, and many hasty judgments of my own, you might want to wait before writing the speakers off so quickly. Things may not be as they first appear, and it's surprising what we can learn if we keep our minds open."

Dr. Davis was obviously embarrassed and his reddened face visibly showed his discomfort. "Yes, sir, you're right. I'll give it a chance. Thank you, sir."

The auditorium quickly began to fill. The general noise subsided as the moderator began the introductions of the day's two lecturers. "Dr. Kevin Soden has been an emergency room physician for almost twenty-five years and now serves as a consultant in occupational medicine to several Fortune 500 companies. He's also a national medical reporter for NBC News and can be seen on NBC's *Today* show.

"Dr. Doug Newburg is a sports psychologist by training and has worked with surgical residents and medical students for over a decade at the University of Virginia. He has interviewed over 350 world-class performers in various fields in his effort to develop his theory on peak performance in medicine. They are here today to bring you a new paradigm for approaching our patients. They've asked me not to waste your time reviewing more of their very impressive credentials because you're likely to forget most of them anyway. What they'd like for you to do instead is actually concentrate on their message, and its potential impact on the practice of medicine." Turning to the two speakers, the introducing doctor said, "Doctors, they're all yours."

I rose to my feet and immediately placed a multicolored baseball cap with a propeller on top of my head. "This is my thinking hat and I'm going to see how well you as an audience can give me the titles for the pictures on my slides." The group quickly got into the game and provided some very funny answers to the slides shown them. Immediately, the audience knew this was not going to be the usual Grand Rounds presentation.

I continued, giving the audience a smile. "I show you these slides because I want you to begin thinking out of the box. I want you approaching prevention in a most unusual way. Why? Because the current model just *isn't* working. Look at

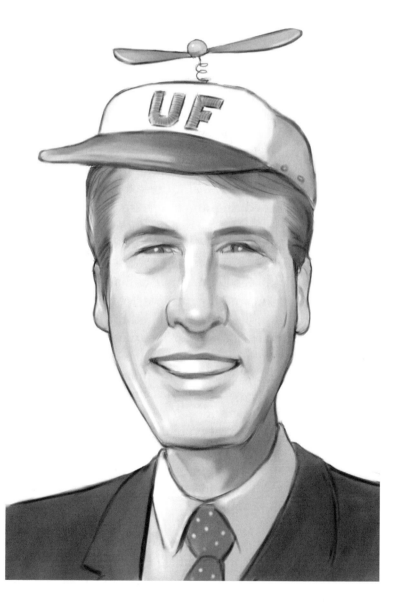

how much effort we currently put into smoking cessation, nutrition and diet counseling, blood pressure reduction and cancer screening programs. Do you think we're really seeing our patients change their habits in response to all those efforts? Unfortunately, the answer must be very, very rarely.

"Let's look at another area of medicine that isn't working as well as it could, either. When you go in to see a patient, or when you yourself go see a doctor, what's usually the first question that's asked? It's commonly some variant of 'What's wrong with you today?' Physicians have done that for years. They've focused on sickness, on ill health, on disease. I'm going to suggest to you today that we need to change the model, the paradigm of medicine, and instead focus on wellness or health with a capital 'H.' The real question needs to be to all of us, 'What's right with you?' We need to look at what makes our patients feel good about themselves—and their lives—and how they can keep getting more of that.

"So here's the key question that we need to ask all of our patients, and ourselves. **'When you felt the best, what was happening in your life?'** I want your answer to focus on what kinds of activities or events were occurring in their lives, or your lives, when you felt the most alive, the most energized about life. It was those times when you felt like leaping out of bed in the morning. You were so energized that you could hardly wait to get your day started. I'm not asking about your cholesterol, your blood sugar, or your bank account necessarily. I want to know about when you felt like all the planets were aligned and most things were going your way. Take a minute now. Think about the question and then write your answer on a piece of paper. You can share your thoughts with your neighbor, or keep them to yourself."

The lecture hall began immediately to buzz with the noise of notebooks being opened and conversation on the assignment. Doctors weren't used to doing this sort of exercise and weren't sure where I was headed.

After a couple of minutes, I continued, "We've all heard of David Letterman's 'Top 10' lists so I thought I'd use that idea to give you the survey results from various groups when asked the same question you were: 'When you felt the best, what was going on in your life?' Here they are:

Top 10 Factors Contributing to Wellness

10. **Time and Space Alone**—Psychologists, psychiatrists, spiritual advisors, and various self-help books all advise us on the need to get away. We all need time to reflect, to meditate and to put our days and our lives into perspective. In our extremely busy society, we have often lost this time to reflect.

9. **Contact with Nature**—Thoreau, in his famous book about Walden Pond, speaks to the need to commune with nature. Why are so many office buildings now built with open spaces and beautiful plantings? Why do we all feel so inspired after being at the beach, in the mountains or in the wide-open spaces? Nature helps to put things into perspective.

8. **Experience Creativity**—We all love to do things that spark our creative sides. It can be in music, the arts, home decorating and even sports. We in medicine do it all the time when we look for creative ways to communicate and relate to patients.

7. **Optimistic State of Mind**—It's the power of positive thinking that separates the above-average performers from the average. The ability to visualize a positive result and to wake up every day and look for the positive makes all the difference. Attitude is everything. It's about the power of intention.

6. **Balanced Nutrition**—You notice I didn't say so many fat grams or serving sizes. People felt the best when they ate a variety of foods. Think of the old saying from

Roman times, 'All things in moderation.' It's only when we eat to excess or neglect certain groups of food that we get in trouble physically.

5. **Work Satisfaction**—You notice people didn't say being in top management or even making a certain amount of money. They talked about feeling good about what they did, day in and day out. When I worked in the ER, I always felt the best when I knew I'd made a difference in those I'd seen. It's not about what you do, but about how you feel when you do it.

4. **Goal Accomplishment**—We all need something to work for. Stephen Covey in his famous book, *The 7 Habits of Highly Effective People,* says, 'Start with the end in mind.' We have to have a vision of what we want. Why do businesses of all sizes set goals for all employees? They all need a goal or a vision to work toward. If there were no single focus, then it would be like a tug of war in which everyone's pulling in different directions. You'll never get much accomplished.

3. **Positive Self-Image**—Does anyone here really like being around people who are always negative? If you don't like yourself, it's difficult to like others and for them to like you. Work on small successes to build that inner confidence that we all need.

2. **Ability to Perform Physical Activities**—You notice that I didn't say here that it was the ability to run a mile in a certain time or to do a set number of push-ups. All that people of all ages wanted was the ability to be physically capable of doing what he or she wanted to do. This was especially true of the elderly. Prevention of cardiovascular disease may push aerobics but the average person only cares about being able to do enough to accomplish his or her goals.

"Now, my final slide, the **#1** factor contributing to a person's state of wellness:

1. **Fulfilling Relationships**—Think about all the times when you had special people in your life and you were really connected to them. The world could hardly be better. Work automatically seemed better, as did every other part of your life. Everything seemed to be right in your universe and it took a lot for other problems to disrupt the happiness that the relationship brought to you."

I then walked even more closely to the audience and said, "I know that what I've presented to you is probably very different from what you expected. It's a paradigm that we currently don't use but I strongly urge you adopt. Any questions?"

An older faculty member sitting close to the front raised his hand and stood up. "What you've presented today is very different from the usual way we discuss prevention and wellness with our patients, but after hearing you, it makes a lot of sense. It reminds me of what one of the fathers of cardiology, Dr. Paul Dudley White, used to talk about. He wanted those of us who trained under him to care for only three parts of our patients—the mind, the body and the spirit. He said if we did that, we'd always connect with our patients and would be addressing their total health. I believe what you're urging us to do is exactly what he had in mind."

I smiled before replying, "I'm humbled, sir. You are absolutely correct. What I want everyone here to consider is not just focusing on someone's cholesterol, or his blood pressure or her weight, but instead doing a better job of focusing on his social history, work history, and family history. Only then will you really connect with your patients."

I glanced at the clock on the side of the lecture hall and then said, "I'm going to stop for now and allow Dr. Newburg his time in front of you. He's going to challenge you as well. He'll give you another reason for learning more about the dreams and goals of your patients, but only if you really want to connect with your patients in a very special relationship. Dr. Newburg."

Dr. Newburg was an outstanding high school and collegiate basketball player and still looked like he could step on the court and play with anyone. He walked with the easy grace of an athlete and appeared comfortable in front of audiences. "Pleasure to be here today. I've worked with a lot of medical students over the last ten years at the University of Virginia and it's always fascinated me to learn what the real dreams are that drive every person's journey to medical school. I'd like to ask each of you to take a moment now and revisit the question, 'Why did you come to medical school?'"

The Student immediately thought to himself. *Where is this guy headed? I know why I went to med school—for the money and the prestige an MD degree gives you. I'm just like Cuba Gooding, Jr. in the movie* Jerry McGuire, *'Show me the money.' Why else would someone go through all this? Who's he kidding? Buy a vowel and get a clue. I'll bet if he asked most of the other people in my class, they'd be here for the same reasons.*

Dr. Newburg interrupted his thoughts with yet another interesting statement. "Health is not about prevention, but totally about preparation. Health is the tool that allows you do what you want to do in life. It goes right back to the factors mentioned by Dr. Soden. The number two factor in wellness was having the physical ability to do the things you wanted to do. You have to be prepared to meet life, to be engaged in what you do every day, and your health allows you to do this. I believe that the most basic question for everyone is 'How do you want to feel each day?' or "What do you like to do that energizes you, that recharges your batteries? You there in the first row, what is it that gets you excited, that you're passionate about?"

The Student couldn't believe that the lecturer had picked him out of the crowd, and visibly reddened despite his best efforts to prevent it. He stood and decided to go for broke. He figured he had nothing to lose, and the excitement in his voice could be heard immediately as he began to answer the question. "I love the movies. I love watching them and I love making my own. It's the classic old flicks that I really like. I can spend hours watching all sorts of flicks. I have a collection of over 200 videos. My movie making just sort of happened when I was in high school. I had to do a project for a class so I decided to do it using my video camera. It just sort of came to me naturally, and I found that I loved it. I guess it's the only real passion I have. If I had to do it all over again, I think I'd like to get into the movie business in some way."

"Thank you," Dr. Newburg replied. "That was a very courageous and honest answer. We all should have a life outside of medicine and there's no reason why both things can't be combined. Just because you become a doctor doesn't mean you can't be in some part of show business. Look at Dr. Michael Crichton who not only writes, but also has been intimately involved in many movies. One of the writers who helped to develop the hit TV show, *ER*, Dr. Joel Baer, is now a pediatric resident. There are also hundreds of physicians doing medical reporting on radio and TV, both nationally and locally. There's even the National Association of Medical Communicators for all those who work in movies, TV and other areas of the media reporting on health-related issues. So if this is truly a dream of yours, don't give it up yet."

Dr. Newburg roamed the stage for a minute before continuing. "Contrary to what the popular press may portray, or what many patients may believe, most physicians do NOT enter medicine for the money. I would argue that the dreams that bring young men and women to medical school are primarily related to their desire to help people. They really enter medicine for the 'emotional income' that they get from caring for their patients. Physicians enter medicine for that fantastic feeling they get when they connect with their patients and make a real positive difference in their lives. If you think about it, it's almost a 'Catch 22' kind of situation. Doctors can't get the 'emotional income' that they really want and need from patients unless they learn how to establish a good doctor-patient relationship. This is the real root cause of a great deal of the frustration and anxiety in medicine today. Many doctors haven't yet learned this simple truth that patients are an integral part of their achieving their own dreams.

"I'm here today to help all of you 'revisit your dreams,' not to mention teaching you how to help your patients find their dreams. Before we get into this too deeply, I want to warn you about one thing. Don't confuse dreams with goals. Your dream is how you want to feel each day when you're engaged in the actual living of your life. Your goal is the actual preparation and work that you must do to achieve your dream. I know it's confusing, so let me tell you a story about a friend of mine, Jeff Rouse. Jeff won a gold medal in swimming in the 1996 Olympics. His goal was to win an Olympic gold medal but his dream was to prepare himself to compete at the highest level of competition in the world. His dream was that wonderful feeling he got when he was competing in events or actually playing to win at some meet. Obtaining his goal was the icing on the cake because he achieved his dream by just competing as best as he could. Now, what happens when you obtain a goal? You always have to set a new goal."

Dr. Newburg got more animated as he spoke and the entire audience could sense his passion about the subject. "I know you're all probably sitting there wondering 'What does this have to do with my patients and me, and the whole subject of wellness?' Actually, I think it's fairly simple. First, let's talk about your dreams as doctors. I think we'd all agree that your goals were or are to become doctors with some sort of specialty. What your dream is—what gets you engaged and gives you those good feelings inside is taking care of people and making a difference in their lives. The key question is: How do you sustain yourself and not get burned out in the midst of the long hours, the constant demands on your time, the hassles of managed care and the dreariness of all the paperwork required today? The answer to this question is by revisiting your dream and reminding yourself that it's the patients who give you energy. So you recharge your batteries by connecting with patients on a deep, personal level. You make the time to really listen to their stories so that you can make a significant difference in their lives. Only then will you keep your dream alive. You have to go back and refocus on what brought you here, and not all the other crap that interferes with our dreams.

"Let me tell you a story about a famous baseball player who happened to be a very good pitcher. It was a very close ball game at the end of an extremely tight pennant race where every game was key to the team's ultimate goal of getting back to the World Series. It was early in this pitcher's career so he was very nervous and getting tighter as the game went on. The manager could see that this young pitcher was getting tentative and the other team was beginning to hit his pitches more solidly. His relief pitchers were worn out so he had to keep the kid in the game. He finally called a time-out and went out to the pitcher's mound to speak to him. He asked the young man, 'Do you know why you've been so successful this season?' 'Because I have a great team behind me,' he replied. 'Yes, that's correct, but you also have done something all season long that's helped you to win. When you got in tight spots, you always challenged the hitter with your best pitch, your fastball. You never backed down. They had to hit your best in order to win. You're not doing that now. You're becoming tentative. What I want you to do is forget everything but what got you here today. Go with what "brung" you. Go with the heat. Throw your fastball, and make them hit your best.' The young kid did and they won that day. Eventually, they went on to win the World Series. What's the point of all that? What 'brung' you to medical school was your desire to help people, so go with it. Don't fight it. Enjoy it and get engaged in it, and look for every opportunity to enjoy your dream by spending time to learn about your patients as much as possible.

"Now, how does this relate to your patients? Every patient also has a dream, just like each of us does. Your job is simple and difficult at the same time. You have to get them to tell you their dream and their goals. Then you can work together with them by getting them in the best possible mental, physical and emotional state of health so that they can do the hard preparatory work that's needed to achieve their dream.

"My friend, Dr. Curt Tribble, the cardiothoracic surgeon who teaches at the University of Virginia, has his coronary bypass patients think about what their dreams are prior to, during and after surgery. It helps them to relax and to focus on those things that bring energy to their lives. It's often the simplest things, like playing with their grandchildren, going fishing, playing a musical instrument or walking on the beach with a loved one. It's these things that bring meaning to our lives, help put life into perspective for us and help to recharge our batteries.

"One of the studies that Erik Erickson has done is to quantify the amount of time it takes to become a world class performer, or WCP. He found that it took almost ten years or 10,000 hours to master a particular profession. It takes many years of extremely hard work to reach the pinnacle of these

WCPs' chosen field of interest, whether it is music, business, medicine or athletics. All of you here today know the time it takes to become a WCP in medicine. You are lucky if it **only** takes ten years of your life. To keep your dream alive during all these periods of ups and downs, you have to constantly revisit your dream, so you can maintain the energy needed to keep you going while you are doing the actual preparatory work. The fun is in the competing and the playing to win, and not necessarily in attaining the actual goal. If achieving the goal of being a doctor is the final end, then we'd have no unhappy doctors—and we all know that's not the case."

Dr. Newburg walked toward the audience again in quest of another volunteer. He singled out one of the residents. "Have you ever heard the terms 'flow' or being 'in the zone'?"

The resident hesitated for a few seconds and then answered, "I'm not sure what 'flow' means but being 'in the zone' is a term that athletes often use when they talk about how they felt during an unusually outstanding athletic performance. I've heard Andre Agassi use the term in tennis, Michael Jordan in basketball and Tiger Woods in golf."

"Great! That's perfect," Dr. Newburg exclaimed. "The 'zone' is the term most often used by athletes while jazz musicians call it being 'in the groove.' 'Flow' is another term for the same things, as well as the name of an excellent book on the subject written by Mihaly Csikszentmihalyi. All these terms have several key features in common. First, you focus intensely on the task or job at hand. Second, time becomes non-existent when you are focused. Time either speeds up so that you don't even realize hours have passed, or it slows down so that you feel ahead of everyone or everything around you. Third, you perform at your highest level—a peak performance, so to speak. Fourth, your focus is so intense that you forget those around you. Michael Jordan would often be unaware of the noise and the people around

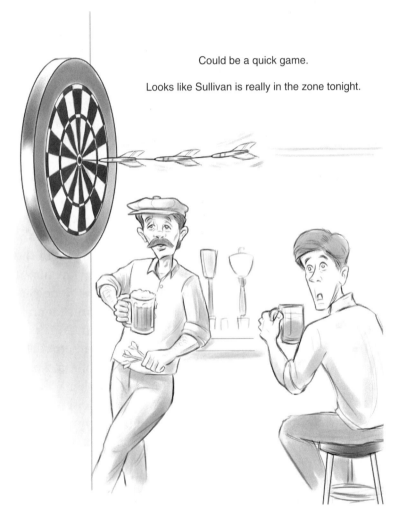

him. Fifth, work seems almost effortless. It seems as if you are exerting very little effort, yet accomplishing so much. Sixth, you find tremendous satisfaction in what you are doing and a real connection to whatever it is you are doing. Finally, when you are done, you feel a deep sense of satisfaction and achievement. Ring a bell with you? Ever had this experience?"

The resident gave Dr. Newburg a huge smile and said, "Yeah, I have. Now it makes so much sense. I never knew it was the same thing that athletes experience, but it felt exactly as you describe it." By then the resident was moving his hands enthusiastically. "I went in to see a woman who was dying the other day to talk about her pain. She began talking about her life, and I could see her face light up as she told me about the things that had meaning to her. I didn't have to say much but just listened. Over an hour went by but it felt like minutes. We were both engaged and knew we had just experienced something special. It was probably the best experience I've had since college, and frankly, it was better than actually learning or doing some new procedure."

"Would you like to experience that feeling again?"

"Damned right I would. Ah, oops, sorry," the resident said with embarrassment.

"Not a problem," laughed Dr. Newburg. "Everyone who's ever enjoyed 'flow' or been in the 'zone' would love to be able to experience it again regularly. I've interviewed hundreds of world-class performers in their fields—athletes, musicians, surgeons, writers and businessmen. Every single one of them has experienced what you have but they've found the secret to recreating this 'zone,' 'flow' or 'resonance'—my own term for this—on a more consistent basis than most other people. That's what makes them great at what they do and energizes them in their work. Dr. Tribble experiences this quite often when performing surgery. He tells me that he gets so focused that he forgets about everything except the surgery in front of him, and many times, doesn't notice that hours have gone by in what seems like minutes."

Dr. Newburg paused for a moment, leaned back with his hands behind his head and said to the group, "I bet some of you are wondering what all this has to do with you and your careers in medicine, aren't you?"

Oh, you can bet your sweet ass on that one. Firm grasp of the obvious on your part, laughed the Student to himself.

Dr. Newburg smiled and leaned toward the audience as if to draw them into the conversation more deeply. "Many of you are just getting started in medicine and in less than two years, you're going to have to choose a residency and a specialty to practice for the rest of your life. What the advisors in this room and I have seen are too many people who've chosen careers for the wrong reasons. As a result, they become very unhappy, get burned out and they just don't enjoy what they do on a daily basis. With all the demands that medicine will put on you, I want all of you to learn how to tune in to yourself and identify those things within medicine that energize you—that give you that feeling of being in the 'zone' or having resonance. It's all about building **your** dream. If you can find resonance in your life, you'll have more and more of those experiences that put you in the 'zone' or provide the feeling of 'flow.' What I try to do with all of my medical students, and with those I see in my consulting work, is provide them a model that will enhance resonance in their lives and for following their dreams, and not someone else's. Only then will you find peace and happiness. If you are happy in what you do, your patients will sense this, and you'll be better for them as well."

Dr. Newburg could see confusion on many people's faces but continued nevertheless, "I know these aren't easy concepts, since most of the world around you is so focused on getting to the top and obtaining material things. What I've found with all my research is that the happiest and most successful people have more than that. They have found a way to incorporate their dreams into their work and into their everyday lives. This is what I'd like to see happen to each of you as well. Thanks for your attention today."

✢ *Perspectives for Doctors* ✢

Why does it take a heart attack or some other serious medical problem to get our attention and get us to change our destructive behaviors? Why can't we make healthy choices in life without having to get a "wake-up call?" When I was on the Cardiology service, I used to see so many people who were on the edge of death from a heart attack and then rallied to a point that they knew they were going to survive. Many were smokers or were very overweight or hadn't exercised in years. One thing that they all had in common was that they said that their heart attacks had finally gotten their attention. Almost universally, they would say that now they would stop smoking, or lose weight or begin exercising. Nothing like being in the jaws of death to get your attention. But why does it have to be that way? Maybe it's the way we approach the whole subject of wellness.

Looking at wellness or total health as a mixture of mind-body-spirit is a marked departure from what many people might answer if asked the definition of each. The World Health Organization defines health as "the complete physical, psychological and social well-being of an individual." The concepts discussed above are part of a new paradigm for medicine—a new way of getting to understand the total health of the whole person. It's what many people call "Holistic Medicine."

Why is there such a need for this kind of approach to medicine and life? When people were asked to define wellness, they often said it's the absence of disease. I challenge that definition for many reasons. Does it mean that you are feeling "healthy" or great about life when your blood pressure is under control, your total cholesterol, triglycerides and LDL, or bad cholesterol, are all within normal and your weight is excellent based on the Metropolitan Life tables? Of course not! It's absurd when you even think about it. It's our mental, emotional and spiritual sides that have just as much of an impact on our "health" or how we feel. Any one of these things can alter our state of total health or wellness. This is why the model of health has to change.

The current (I would argue old) paradigm for prevention in medicine has long focused on those diseases or problems that conform to certain rules. First, the medical problems that can be considered preventable must be identifiable with a relatively easy-to-use test, such as measuring blood pressure, doing a Pap smear, having a mammogram or getting a blood test. Second, there must be a number of people who have this problem or disease so that screening for it becomes cost effective. Rare diseases do not fall under this paradigm. Third, by identifying the disease early enough before major damage has been done, treatment can have an impact on long-term health by preventing problems down the road. Fourth, the test must be good enough to have both few false positives and few false negative results. These rules deal strictly with physical disease, such as breast cancer, high blood pressure, cholesterol and diabetes. This is important, and I don't mean to downplay this model of wellness or prevention, but they don't address the problems of the inner self that make up so much of how we feel about life in general, as in the story above. Clearly, the old model works to a degree but it requires constant education, is costly and only seems to reach a small handful of people who really could be helped by it.

Let's consider the same question asked in the lecture above: "**When you felt the best, what was going on in your life?**" I'll take a bet that when you felt the best was not necessarily when you had the most money or the most security. It might have been when you were in school learning a profession, or maybe when you were struggling early in a career, or it even might have been the time when your kids were young and your house was crazy at times. It didn't matter that you didn't have all the best things in life or you ate fast food or didn't get to exercise everyday. Rather, it was being creative, having goals and feeling the excitement of wonderful relationships. That is real wellness.

Dr. Doug Newburg is very real and is sincerely committed to helping people find their dreams. He has developed a unique easy-to-understand model for helping people get what they want out of life. He has written numerous articles on the subject and is currently working on a series of books to help people gain "resonance" in their lives. He defines resonance as that balance between the external demands of the material world and our own internal dreams that bring us peace and total health.

While studying to get his Ph.D. in sports psychology, Dr. Newburg interviewed over 250 world-class performers to see if he could find the common thread that made them achieve as they had. He found that all shared a few things in common. They all were engaged in what they were doing when they were preparing for the goal they wanted to achieve. They were all committed to preparing as best as possible for winning at what they did. They might not win, but they prepared to compete at the highest levels and they played to win. They knew that some things were out of their control so they had to prepare themselves to expect obstacles, and then deal with them as they came along. All they could do was to physically and mentally prepare themselves to do the best they could, and then let the chips fall where they may. Out of all this research, Dr. Newburg developed a simple model or process for achieving resonance (his term) in every person's life.

6 Steps to Achieving Your Dream (Resonance)

1. <u>How do you want to feel each day?</u>—World-class performers know that they help to create how they want to feel everyday. You have to decide and then act that way. Positive people act positively. People who want to be engaged with others look for opportunities to connect with people. Each of us must take responsibility for how we want to feel, and then act that way.

2. <u>How do I make that feeling happen?</u>—This is the preparation phase of achieving your dream. You have to take time at the end of each day to review when you felt best, who helped you to feel that way and what added to or took away from that feeling of engagement in your life. With this information you can create the kind of environment that fosters the positive feelings that you want to create. Stay focused on the things you can control and go for it.

3. <u>What gets in the way of or takes away the feeling?</u>—Obstacles and people are a part of everyone's life. Many of them are out of our control, but you can choose how you respond to them. World-class performers know they will experience obstacles but they learn how to focus on getting back the good feeling of engagement in life. They know what they can control to help get those feelings back again.

4. <u>How do I get back the feelings I want?</u>—Everyone is different. What makes me feel good and refocused on what's important is my family. I think about the laughter and the special gifts that each of my five kids brings to me and I immediately smile again. Sometimes just digging down and solving a problem is enough to stimulate me and get me engaged again. The satisfaction of doing and not letting someone or something beat me down is positive enough.

5. <u>What are you really willing to work for?</u>—Many people can tell you their dreams but when the real work is needed, there's just no follow-through. If you aren't willing to do the work, then you won't get the feelings you want. Only you can take responsibility for this. You can't blame the lack of hard work on anyone but yourself. Pick carefully and only choose feelings and outcomes that you are willing to work for.

6. <u>Time to revisit your dream?</u>—As you achieve certain successes and failures, it helps to revisit your dream to make sure it's the right one for you. Many people work hard to achieve a certain goal or dream and then once they get it, realize it's not for them. By revisiting your dream, you re-engage in the process and remember why you picked the dream you did. If it takes ten years to get to certain dreams, you have to revisit or you'll lose the energy and focus needed to keep you performing each day.

"Revisiting your dream," reminds me of my own very long, extremely circuitous path to medical school and to where I am today. I believe it demonstrates the importance of taking stock and why revisiting your dream can change your life.

Despite having athletic scholarships to some very good schools, I attended a small Catholic, liberal arts College in North Carolina—Belmont Abbey College. I had serious aspirations of being a Catholic monk (not the kind who don't talk). I wanted to do something to help people and feel like I was making a difference in people's lives. The monk vocation was put on hold after I realized that playing sports was so important to me at that time in my life. I decided to become a history major because it was the first major open when I registered as a junior. I knew that I wasn't smart enough to be a science major. As I neared graduation, I knew that I wanted to coach and work in a college or university. It would be intellectually stimulating and I'd get to help people.

Toward this end I went to graduate school to get a degree in personnel administration in higher education. This experience helped me to realize that I had the brains to do more advanced educational work and that I needed competitive challenges in my life to feel engaged and energized. As I gained confidence in myself, I again wanted to do more to help people. As I revisited my grad school dream, I realized in my gut that this wasn't the long-term profession for me. I had some college friends who were in medical school and talked enthusiastically about how exciting and challenging it was. So, you guessed it, I decided to apply to medical school despite having NO science courses at this point. I started taking some while in grad school and did very well. Therefore I returned to my undergraduate school, Belmont Abbey, and took all my science in one year while working as the Assistant Dean of Students. I took the Medical College Admission Test without science courses and did miserably in the science portion but very well in the other sections. Fortunately, a few schools decided to offer me a spot anyway. As a result, I ended up at the University of Florida College of Medicine. It was one of the best decisions of my life. The people at the school were great and I'd found the intellectual challenge that I needed, plus I was fulfilling my desire to help people. I had finally found a home.

My residency was in Family Practice but again I realized that I liked the excitement of something else. The ER met my need for excitement and constant challenges so I ended up working in local Charlotte, North Carolina area emergency rooms. I had found my niche. I ended every long, busy shift energized and feeling like I had made a difference. I haven't looked back since. If I hadn't taken time along my life journey to take stock, to assess my dreams, then I might not have been willing to take risks. I knew I wasn't happy at times and that I needed to change what I was doing or I'd be miserable. Whenever I tune in and follow my gut, I don't go wrong. Dr. Newburg will tell you that the same thing will work for you as well.

Finally, feeling good and maintaining your health is all about choices. You are the one who will make the choices that will have the most significant impact on your life. Staying healthy is a choice and there are a number of choices that will allow you to take charge of your life.

Take stock every day. Tune in to how you're feeling. Pay special attention to those people and things that provide energy in your life and that get you engaged in living. Take action based on what your dreams and goals are. Then revisit your dreams periodically to help keep you focused and provide the energy needed to keep you working toward the goals you've set.

Taking Your Pulse

The Jar of Life

A philosophy professor stood before his class and had some items in front of him. When class began, he picked up a large empty mayonnaise jar and proceeded to fill it with 2-inch-diameter rocks, right to the top.

He then asked the students if the jar was full. They agreed that it was.

So the professor then picked up a box of pebbles and poured them into the jar. He shook the jar lightly so that the pebbles could fill the open areas between the rocks. The students laughed.

He asked his students again if the jar was full. They agreed that yes, it was.

The professor then picked up a box of sand and poured it into the jar. The sand filtered down and filled up everything else.

"Now," said the professor, "I want you to recognize that this is your life. The rocks are the important things—your family, your partner, your health, and your children—anything that is so important to you that if it were lost, you would be destroyed. The pebbles are the other things in life that matter, but on a smaller scale. The pebbles are things like your house, your job and your car. The sand is everything else: the small stuff.

"If you put the sand or the pebbles into the jar first, there is no room for the rocks. The same goes for your life. If you spend all your energy and time on the small stuff, on material things, you will never have room for the things that are truly most important.

"Pay attention to the things that are critical in your life. Play with your children. Take time to get medical checkups. Take your partner out dancing. There will always be time to go to work, clean the house, give a dinner party and fix the disposal.

"Take care of the rocks first, the things that matter most. Set your priorities. The rest are just pebbles and sand."

Graduation from medical school was less than two weeks away and the Advisor had asked the Student to come to his office again for what would be their last formal meeting. The Student was on his final rotation, so technically there wasn't anything more that the Advisor needed to do. He had had two years to make his impact on his advisee so only time would tell what that would be. The other reason the Advisor had asked the Student to come to his office was to find out what the results of Match Day were. Every year on Match Day all fourth-year students in all U.S. medical schools learned for the first time where they would be doing their residency training. It was a day like no other for all medical students—a day of great joy for most, but a time of considerable heartache for those who failed to match in any program.

The Advisor had been out of country for two months teaching overseas and preferred not to know the results of the Student's match until he heard it for himself. The Student had been quite clear from their first contact of his interest in radiology, and the Advisor had sent letters of recommendation to three good, solid radiology residency programs. When the Student finally got to his office, they exchanged pleasantries briefly before the Advisor could contain himself no more. "Well, don't keep me in suspense, which residency program is going to be lucky enough to get you next year?"

"I'm going to be at Carolinas Medical Center in Charlotte. It's got one of the best programs in the country, and I was unbelievably lucky to get in at the last minute."

"Carolinas Medical Center? What are you talking about? I never wrote a letter of recommendation for that program. They don't even have a radiology program." The Advisor was clearly taken aback and his total confusion was obvious in both his face and in voice.

The Student had a huge grin on his face as he answered with great glee. "I know they don't have a radiology program. I'm going into Family Practice."

The Advisor had been standing up until this point but quickly sat back in his chair. "Family Practice? You're going into Family Practice? You're the guy who wanted the green—the money. You wanted to avoid too much time with patients. What happened to all that?" the Advisor said incredulously.

It was the Student's turn to laugh now before speaking. "You're right. When I first came to you, I was all gung-ho for radiology. I didn't care about anything else, and maybe I didn't even care much about anyone else . . . except me. Many things have happened to me during these past two years that slowly got under my skin and ate at my subconscious, until I knew this was the only way to go for me. All the teachers who taught me all about communicating with patients and listening to their stories finally got to me. I found that I began to enjoy hearing their stories, and that I was good at getting people to talk to me. I began to take pride in taking a good history and being able to show up some of the residents, especially when it came to knowing our patients. I did my family practice rotation with Dr. Walker and my medicine rotation with Dr. Porter, Dr. Bianchi and Dr. Justice. Those docs taught me so much and helped me to see such a different side of medicine. I tried to fight it and did so . . . right up until the end. I applied for the residency in radiology but took my name out of the hat while you were gone. Dr. Hill had to use all his considerable pull to get me the residency slot in Charlotte when one of their first-year picks dropped out at the last minute due to a personal situation. I guess I really surprised you, didn't I?" the Student said with a huge smile.

The Advisor never used strong language but was so shocked that he did then. "You're damned right you did. I never saw this one coming . . . and I thought I was good at reading people. I go away for a little while and you decide to go crazy. Unbelievable! And, why family practice and not medicine?"

"Fair question. I kind of vacillated between medicine and family practice but I knew that I wanted primary care. I wanted to be on the front lines interacting with patients every day. You know, I actually came to like kids. I also liked the idea of being able to treat the whole family rather than just the adults, and I wanted that long-term relationship with my patients. Do you know one of the first things you ever said that stuck with me and really impacted the way I began to look at what I did in medicine?"

Now it was the Advisor's turn to act totally dumb and have to say, "I have no idea."

"The first time I met with you in your office you mentioned the term 'emotional income.' It was that thing—that feeling we got from our patients that energized us—that kept us going, even on our bad days. When I really took the time to look inside and examine myself, to listen to what my gut was telling me, I realized that every time I truly interacted with a patient, I got that emotional income. When I took the time to listen to my patients, I realized that I became ramped, buzzed, turned on. It was incredible!" The Student laughed. "The other thing that impressed me while doing my family practice rotation with Dr. Walker was the friendship that he developed with his patients over time. With many of his patients, he became 'family' to them . . . and they with him. I really liked and wanted the chance to experience some of that myself. I realized that it was all a part of what you had been trying to help me see."

The Advisor leaned closer to the Student and began to speak. "Thank you for that wonderful compliment. It means more than you'll ever know. This kind of experience is what teaching and interacting with students and residents is all about. You were obviously open to looking at things in a different way, and that's a compliment to you. I'm just happy that you've found those things that energize you and bring you joy. It's not always easy to sustain that, so the key is being open to new experiences and new things that will help you grow for the rest of your life. Just take the time to tune in to what your gut is telling you. If you do, you'll always move in the right direction and you'll always be true to the dream that lives in your heart." The Adviser paused for a minute, just staring at the Student. "Do you mind if I share a few thoughts with you before you go?"

"No, of course not," the Student laughed. "You've never been shy before so why start now?"

The Advisor had to grin at that last remark as well. "You so shocked me today that I'm not my usual self. You know, I've made a lot of mistakes over my sixty-plus years, but luckily, I've had even more successes. There are some things that I'd like you to think about as you go about your life, and the practice of medicine. Do you know that the practice of medicine provides both the greatest gift to us as well as the greatest tragedy? Do you know what these might be?"

"No, I can't say that I do," the Student replied with a curious look on his face.

"The greatest gift that we get as physicians is the sharing of our patients' lives with us. We learn about their dreams, their hopes, their successes, their failures—and their families. We learn what they did wrong, and what they did right. We see for ourselves every day the effects of lifestyle on people's lives. If our patients choose poor health behaviors, they often suffer adverse health effects down the road. If they choose good health behaviors, then they increase their odds of being able to do the things they want to do in life. Do you agree?"

"Sure," the Student said with a puzzled look on his face. "But, what's the tragedy?"

The Advisor got a rueful smile on his face and shook his head slowly from side to side before replying. "The greatest tragedy is that we are given this wonderful gift—the stories that our patients tell us. We have the opportunity to learn so much, yet we don't seem to take advantage of it. That's the real tragedy. We're not unlike our patients in that regard. Let me give you a perfect example. Physicians see first-hand every day how lifestyle behaviors lead to heart disease, but they themselves refuse to stop smoking, lose weight, take medicine or eat properly until they're at death's door with a heart attack. Why do so many of us fail to take care of ourselves physically, emotionally or spiritually when we can see the terrible results of these same behaviors in our patients?

"To be a doctor, lawyer, pharmacist or any other professional, you have to be extremely focused on your goal for many years and are almost forced to neglect many other things in the process of obtaining those goals. As a general rule, physicians are not very balanced. They're good at science but not much else . . . especially insight into themselves and their emotional state. They often don't take the time to learn much about themselves because they've been so focused on becoming doctors and taking care of people. Why do so many physicians' marriages end up in divorce despite the fact that they can see what not having time with their families does to their patients' spouses and children? They make medicine or whatever their job is their mistress and don't spend the time or the energy to work at the relationships that they say are important. You can say what you want, but we all put our time where our priorities are. The great tragedy is that we just don't seem to take action based on the life story gifts we are given by our patients. We have to make our own mistakes before we learn. It's like watching a train wreck in slow motion and not being able to do something about it. It's so sad. I guess we're no different from anyone else in this regard." The Advisor paused for a minute with his head down peering fixedly at his lap. "Do you know one of the biggest problems that physicians face while in practice?"

The Student thought for a few seconds and replied, "Alcohol and drug use?"

"Good guess, but I think the most common problem I see in my colleagues, and what I hear from other physicians, is burnout. Doctors just get tired of all the crap. They're no longer energized by the practice of medicine. They hate going to the office and they begin to resent their patients. Their patients begin to feel this and leave that physician because they don't like being cared for by an unhappy, non-focused doctor. The physician then gets more upset and his or her unhappiness with the practice of medicine soon becomes a self-fulfilling prophecy. Sometimes these feelings of anger, depression or unhappiness begin to spill over to their families, and then there's no place that the doctor finds any happiness. Fortunately, many physicians realize that something is wrong and step back to examine the problem, or they go ask for help from others. Often this forces some changes in their practice, or they might even end up switching careers. The lesson that we all need to take home from this is that we need to examine our lives regularly, so that we can detect the symptoms of burnout before they begin to cause serious problems. We never want to feel trapped or begin to take our unhappiness out on our patients . . . or our families. *Capisce?*"

The Student nodded his head in understanding.

"A couple of final bits of advice if you hear nothing else of what I've said. Keep your life as simple as possible. This means not taking on huge home mortgages or car payments. Keep your bills and lifestyle in line so that you're not tied to your practice because of monetary 'golden handcuffs.' If you're not careful, your financial responsibilities may leave you no options if you want to switch careers, or cut back to pursue other interests.

"The second bit of important advice is to choose your practice wisely. Look at it as a marriage. You spend more waking hours with your partners in practice then you do with your family. Don't just opt for the big bucks, but look for compatibility and group happiness. If you care for patients in a quality manner in a practice you like, then adequate financial rewards will come, and you'll have all the happiness that medicine can bring."

The Advisor got up and began to walk the Student to the door. "I didn't mean to wax so philosophically but I want your dreams to come true, and I want you to enjoy the practice of medicine as I have for these many years. Being a physician is a gift, and I hope you'll always respect what we've been given. I can't tell you how wonderful it's been for me to share your medical school experience. I thank you for our time together. It's meant so much to me."

The Student couldn't believe what he was hearing. "How can you say that? I'm the one who's learned so much. If you'd have told me two years ago that I'd end up where I

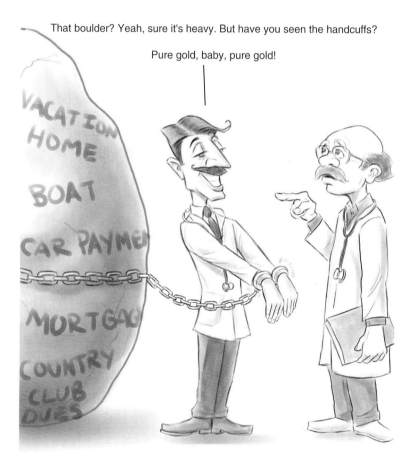

am now, I would have wondered what kind of funny cigarette you'd been smoking. I never saw any of this coming. You know, when I asked some of your previous advisees about you, they wouldn't tell me anything. They just told me to give you a chance. I'm so glad that I did. I'll never forget you," the Student said with great emotion in his voice.

The Advisor put his arms out and hugged the Student. "If you've learned something valuable from me, pass it on so that others will learn as well. Medicine is all about passing the baton. See one, do one, teach one. If you do share what you've learned, it will be the greatest gift you can give me."

And that's just what I've done with you.

Final Thoughts

In two recent surveys of medical professionals, more and more doctors are suffering from the effects of burnout. A 1997 survey of Sacramento, California doctors indicated that 81% of those physicians suffered from medium-to-high levels of burnout. One of the authors of the study, Dr. Martha Snider, reported, "that it is the most idealistic committed doctor who burns out." According to this report, the typical burnout physician is thirty-seven to forty-eight years old, has practiced for four to seven years and is in a multi-specialty group. Interestingly, there was no statistical difference between burnout rates in men and women, nor between primary care doctors and specialists.

Burnout is different than stress. Burnout is more a chronic state with mental and physical exhaustion, loss of perspective, cynicism, frustration, anxiety, depression and, often, the inability to recover from these conditions. Dr. John-Henry Pfifferling, director of the Center for Professional Well-Being in Durham, North Carolina, states, "Ninety percent of the problem is related to environmental factors and the doctor gets into trouble because of the marked disparity between idealized expectations and reality."

The generally acknowledged major causes of burnout today are the incessant demands of medical practice today and the inability to control one's life, especially in the setting of managed care. Managed care organizations (MCOs) have multiplied the hassles of practice, increased paperwork, and made physicians work longer for less pay. Picking the type of practice that fits both personality and needs is one of the most important decisions a physician will make. Picking the wrong practice will almost guarantee unhappy patients and frustrated doctors. The wrong practice situation can even sour a physician on the entire practice of medicine forever. Like divorce in a marriage, leaving a practice situation can be bitter, extremely stressful and have a lifelong impact on the individual involved.

Another major factor contributing to burnout is trying to balance a large practice with family demands. Something eventually has to give if a doctor doesn't set limits and define boundaries. It's very easy to get sucked into believing that you have to save the world, especially when it feeds the ego.

To prevent burnout, a physician must learn to take care of him or herself and make life balance a priority. (Great advice for anyone no matter what who they are and what they do.) Here are some things that each of us can do to take charge of our lives and obtain the happiness we each want.

It's your life and your career. You can take charge, take care and choose happiness. The choice is yours.

10 Ways to Take Charge of Your Life

1. **Always seek a mission in life that is grounded in a higher good and service to others.**
2. **Keep laughter and fun in all you do.**

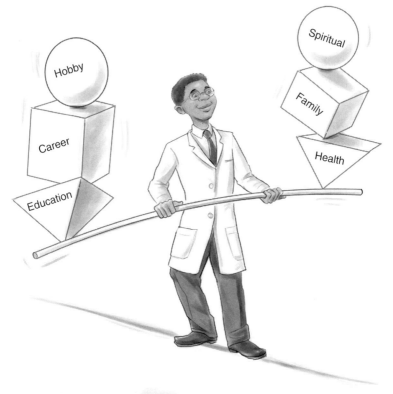

Wow, that doctor has really mastered that balancing act.

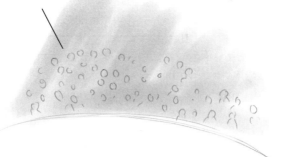

3. Remember "when you felt the best in your life" and work toward keeping those experiences in your life.
4. Exercise regularly and take care of yourself.
5. Remain curious all your life and look for creative outlets.
6. Work at the important relationships in your life every day.
7. Find something you're passionate about and work at it . . . outside the office.
8. Seek balance in your life.
9. Set boundaries and delegate.
10. Regularly examine how you feel emotionally and physically and, if there are problems, take corrective action.

Index